# Understanding
# **Varicose Veins**

Professor Bruce Campbell

Published by Family Doctor Publications Limited
in association with the British Medical Association

**IMPORTANT NOTICE**
This book is intended not as a substitute for personal
medical advice but as a supplement to that advice for
the patient who wishes to understand more about his or
her condition.

Before taking any form of treatment
YOU SHOULD ALWAYS CONSULT YOUR MEDICAL
PRACTITIONER.

In particular (without limit) you should note that
advances in medical science occur rapidly and some
information about drugs and treatment contained in this
booklet may very soon be out of date.

© Family Doctor Publications 2002–2006
Updated 2002, 2003, 2006

Family Doctor Publications, PO Box 4664, Poole, Dorset BH15 1NN

**ISBN: 1 903474 59 0**

# Contents

# About the author

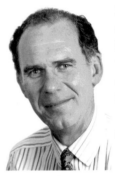

**Professor Bruce Campbell** is a consultant vascular surgeon in Exeter, with wide experience in treating diseases of the arteries and veins, and a particular interest in varicose veins. He has been involved in organising vascular surgery nationally and is well known for his writing and lecturing on vascular disease.

# Introduction

## What are varicose veins?

Varicose veins are very common. They are the lumpy, raised, blue veins that we see on the legs of people wearing shorts, bathing costumes or skirts. Many more people hide their varicose veins by always wearing trousers or thick tights, because they are embarrassed about their appearance.

The veins that become varicose are the ones just under the skin – not the important deeper veins, which carry most of the blood and which can sometimes be affected by dangerous thrombosis (formation of a blood clot). This means that, if varicose veins are troublesome, they can be removed by an operation or sealed off by injection treatment (sclerotherapy).

The demand for varicose vein treatment is huge: more than 50,000 operations are done each year on the National Health Service in England and Wales. Most people with varicose veins never develop serious medical problems (such as ulcers). This means that waiting lists for varicose vein treatment are often long and in many localities the NHS will not fund treatment for people whose varicose veins are not causing problems.

## What varicose veins are not

Veins can be seen forming a pattern under the skin of the legs, particularly in people with pale skin. These are the normal veins that everyone has beneath the skin, but that show up more easily in some people than others. They are not varicose veins unless they become widened, tortuous and bulging.

Spider veins, flare veins and other tiny red or blue veins are also common on the skin of the legs, particularly with increasing age (although a few people develop them when they are young). These are not the same as varicose veins and do not mean that varicose veins are more likely to develop.

## Words used to describe obvious leg veins

Different words have been used to describe and classify the various kinds of veins that can be seen in the legs. There is no universally accepted classification, but the one that is probably best describes:

- 'varicose veins' (wider than four millimetres or mm)
- 'reticular veins' (less than four millimetres wide)
- 'telangiectases' (little veins in the skin less than one millimetre wide – the ones more often called spider veins or flare veins).

There is a system called the Basle classification, which describes 'trunk varices', 'reticular varices' and 'hyphen-webs', but doctors do not usually use these terms.

## The problems caused by varicose veins

Varicose veins often cause no trouble at all. The most usual problem is concern about their appearance: they become prominent on standing because they fill with blood under pressure, but become flat on lying down.

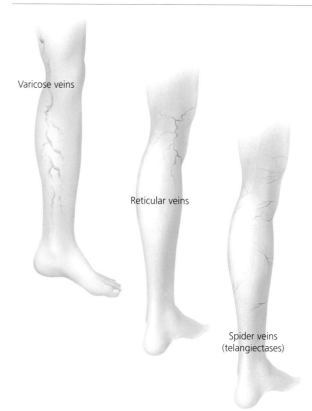

Varicose veins

Reticular veins

Spider veins
(telangiectases)

Different words have been used to describe and classify the various kinds of veins that can be seen in the legs, but there is no universally accepted classification.

Especially after prolonged standing they can cause feelings of heaviness, aching, itching and discomfort. Sometimes varicose veins cause ankle swelling (but other causes are much more common).

In a few people varicose veins eventually lead to eczema and darkening of the skin at the ankle, because of the high blood pressure in the veins there.

Ulcers can then form in the damaged skin. The prospect of ulcers worries a lot of people, but ulcers only ever affect a very small proportion of those with varicose veins, and there are almost always warning signs first. There is no special reason for people with varicose veins and healthy skin to worry about ulceration.

Varicose veins also cause concern about the possibility of clotting or 'thrombosis', but there is little reason for this. The kind of thrombosis that can be dangerous is in the deep veins of the legs – not in the ones under the skin that form varicose veins. Deep vein thrombosis sometimes causes blood clots to pass to the lungs (pulmonary embolism) or leads to permanent leg swelling – this is discussed later in the book. Varicose veins can be affected by thrombophlebitis (they become hard and inflamed), but it is very unusual for this to lead to serious deep vein thrombosis.

Other problems such as bleeding are very rare, and affect only a minute number of people with varicose veins.

It is worth repeating that varicose veins seldom cause serious medical problems of any kind.

## Treatments for varicose veins

As most varicose veins do not cause serious problems, treatment is seldom essential. Aching and heaviness can often be controlled by support stockings or tights. Smaller varicose veins can be dealt with by injections (sclerotherapy) which seal off the veins and make them disappear. Larger ones have traditionally been treated by surgery for a good long-term result, but foam sclerotherapy may also be a reasonable option.

Nowadays specialists investigate the blood flow in the veins by ultrasound. This identifies exactly which veins have valves that are not working properly, and allows for more precise planning of treatment than was possible before. Well-planned and thorough treatment is more likely to provide long-term freedom from varicose veins.

The only reason for considering treatment by injections or surgery is if varicose veins are causing sufficient trouble. For some people, their appearance may be so unacceptable that they want to be rid of their veins for cosmetic reasons alone. In general, discomfort, or a combination of discomfort and cosmetic embarrassment, is the most common reason for people requesting treatment. Fear that varicose veins might get worse, or that ulcers might develop in healthy skin, is not a good reason on its own for having something done.

This book explains how varicose veins can cause trouble, and describes the pros and cons of the different kinds of treatment. A number of different methods for treating varicose veins have become available in recent years and this has made both discussion and the choice of treatment more complex.

## KEY POINTS

■ Varicose veins are very common

■ They seldom cause serious problems

■ Treatment is necessary only if veins are sufficiently troublesome

■ New treatments for varicose veins have made the choice more complex

# All about varicose veins

## Arteries, capillaries and veins

Before talking about varicose veins, it is very important to understand the difference between arteries and veins, and to know something about the normal veins of the legs.

Arteries, capillaries and veins are the tubes that carry blood around the body: they can all be called 'blood vessels'. They are all part of 'the circulation'.

## The arteries

As the heart pumps, it sends blood around the body through the arteries. The arteries branch into smaller and smaller vessels, until the blood flows into capillaries. The walls of capillaries are only one cell thick, so that oxygen, glucose and other substances can pass through them to nourish the tissues. The waste materials of metabolism, such as carbon dioxide and lactic acid, filter in the opposite direction into the capillaries. A network of capillaries runs close to the cells in every part of the body, delivering nutrients and taking away waste products in the bloodstream.

## The circulatory system

A network of capillaries runs close to the cells in every part of the body. The capillaries have very thin walls which allow nutrients to pass through into the tissues and waste products to filter back into the capillaries.

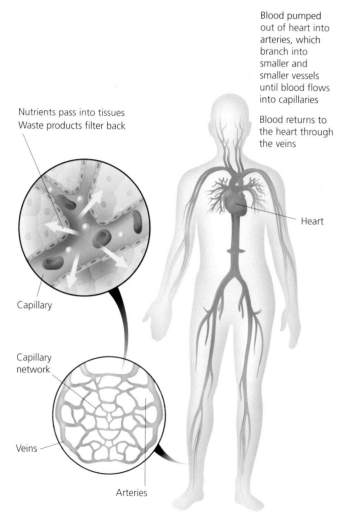

Blood pumped out of heart into arteries, which branch into smaller and smaller vessels until blood flows into capillaries

Blood returns to the heart through the veins

Nutrients pass into tissues
Waste products filter back

Heart

Capillary

Capillary network

Veins

Arteries

## The veins

Capillaries join to form slightly larger vessels (venules, or tiny veins) and these in turn join up to form veins. As more tributaries join each main vein, so it gets wider, and eventually blood returns to the heart through the two largest veins – the superior vena cava from the upper part of the body, and the inferior vena cava carrying blood from the legs, pelvis and abdomen.

Small veins, joining a larger one, are called tributaries (rather than branches) because blood is flowing up them into the larger vein – like water in the tributaries of a large river.

The blood flowing through the veins is darker than the blood in arteries, because it has less oxygen in it. In contrast to blood flow in arteries, the flow in veins is slower and is not pulsatile. In the leg veins, activity of the leg muscles is important in helping to pump blood back to the heart. One-way valves in the veins make the blood flow towards the heart. The valves are particularly important in veins of the legs, because blood could otherwise flow the wrong way (downwards) when we are standing up.

## Diseases of arteries and veins

The common diseases affecting arteries and veins are quite different. 'Atherosclerosis' narrows and blocks arteries, causing heart attacks, strokes and gangrene, but it does not cause problems in the veins. Varicose veins have nothing to do with heart attacks, strokes or amputation of the leg. 'Thrombosis' means clotting of blood in a blood vessel and can occur in either veins or arteries, but the causes and effects are different.

Thrombosis in the deep veins of the legs can be

## The vein system in the leg

The veins in the leg are divided into two systems – the deep veins and the superficial veins. The two systems are linked periodically by perforating veins. A superficial vein can become varicose because a perforating vein is allowing blood to flow the wrong way (outwards).

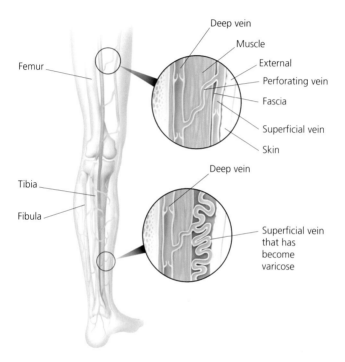

Femur

Deep vein

Muscle

External

Perforating vein

Fascia

Superficial vein

Skin

Tibia

Fibula

Deep vein

Superficial vein that has become varicose

dangerous (see 'Thrombosis, phlebitis and bleeding', page 28), but these veins are different from those forming varicose veins.

## The deep and superficial veins of the legs

The veins of the legs are divided into two systems – the deep veins (which run deep to the leathery layer of fascia surrounding the muscles) and the superficial veins (which run in the layer of fat just beneath the skin). The superficial veins are the ones that you can see (for example, on your foot or around the ankle) and they are the ones that can become varicose.

It is essential to keep in mind these two different systems – deep and superficial – in order to understand varicose veins and their treatment.

## Perforating veins

In a number of places in the leg, the superficial and deep veins are linked by perforating veins (or 'perforators'). They are called perforators because they perforate the leathery fascial layer surrounding the muscles of the legs. Normally their valves should allow blood to flow only inwards – from the superficial veins to the deep veins. If the valves stop working properly, then blood is pushed out into the superficial veins when the muscles contract: this is one reason for high pressure in the superficial veins, and can be a cause of varicose veins.

## Valves in the veins

All the leg veins have delicate valves inside them, which should allow the blood to flow only upwards (towards the heart), or from the superficial veins to the deep ones through the perforating veins. The valves protect against the head of pressure that would otherwise exist in the veins of the legs on standing. If there were no valves, there would be a pressure in the veins at the ankle equivalent to the height of the column of blood all the way up to the heart. It is this head of pressure that causes symptoms and damage when the valves stop working properly, as they often do in varicose veins. A valve occurs every five to ten centimetres in the main superficial veins of the legs.

## The muscle pump

When blood is pumped into the arteries by the heart, it is pushed forwards under high pressure. Only a little of this pressure is left after blood has filtered through the capillaries, to push it through the veins, and the action of the muscles provides a pumping action that helps to push the blood up through the veins. This 'muscle pump' is particularly important in the legs, because when we are standing blood has to travel a long way 'uphill' to get back to the heart.

The deep veins lie within and between the muscles of the calf and thigh. All the muscles are surrounded by a firm leathery layer of 'fascia', so as they contract

## The calf muscle pump

The contraction of muscles compressing veins helps push blood up through the leg veins back to the heart. The valves allow the blood to flow towards the heart only.

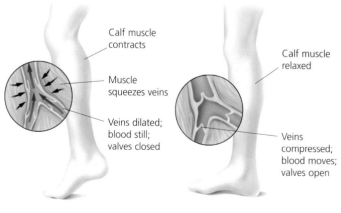

Calf muscle contracts

Muscle squeezes veins

Veins dilated; blood still; valves closed

Calf muscle relaxed

Veins compressed; blood moves; valves open

and relax blood is forced up the deep veins. Normally, the valves in the veins make sure that blood flows only upwards in the deep and superficial veins, and inwards through the perforating veins.

If the valves stop working, then the muscle pump cannot do its job properly. Damaged valves in the deep veins mean that blood is not pumped upwards, and this can be particularly harmful if the veins at knee level are affected. Failure of valves in the perforating veins allows blood to be pushed out under high pressure into the superficial veins, which can lead to varicose veins.

## Soldiers and the muscle pump

Soldiers give us two good examples about how the muscle pump can be helped to work. Have you noticed how soldiers standing to attention for a long time will sway to and fro just slightly? They have been taught to contract and relax their calf muscles so that blood is pumped up their legs, rather than pooling in the calf veins. Particularly on a hot day, when all the veins are wide and dilated, pooling of blood in the leg veins can occasionally make them faint if they do not do this.

The other military lesson about the muscle pump is provided by the puttees that soldiers used to wear, wrapped tightly around their ankles and calves. These formed a firm layer around the whole lower leg (rather like the fascia around the muscles and deep veins) and probably helped the muscle pump to squeeze blood up through the veins during long marches.

## Which veins become varicose?
### The long saphenous vein

This vein and its tributaries are the ones that most often form varicose veins. The long saphenous vein (LSV) is formed from tributaries in the foot, and is visible in many people when they stand, as the vein just in front of the bone on the inner side of the ankle. It runs up the inner side of the calf and the thigh, and at the groin dives to join the main deep vein (the femoral vein).

## The short saphenous vein
This is the other main vein under the skin of the leg, the tributaries of which can become varicose, but it is affected much less often than the LSV. The short saphenous vein (SSV) starts just behind the bone on

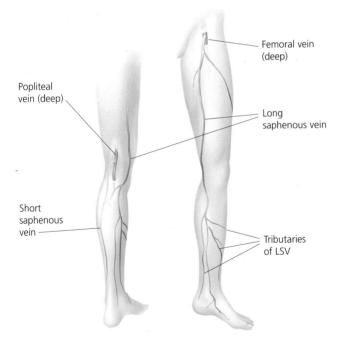

The long saphenous vein (LSV) and its tributaries most often form varicose veins. The short saphenous vein (SSV) and its tributaries can also become varicose but less often.

the outer side of the ankle, and runs up the middle of the back of the calf. It usually dives to join the main deep vein just above and behind the knee (the popliteal vein), but this varies and before any operation on the SSV it needs to be checked by a scan.

It has been suggested that the long saphenous vein should be called the 'great saphenous vein' and the short saphenous vein the 'small saphenous vein'. These alternative names are used in other countries but the names 'long' and 'short' are still usual in the UK, and are used throughout this book.

## Perforating veins

In almost any part of the leg, a perforating vein can develop incompetent valves. This allows blood to be pumped outwards under pressure into superficial veins, causing them to become stretched and varicose.

## Any vein

Any vein under the skin, in any part of the leg, can become varicose, without valve problems in the LSV, SSV or perforating veins. These varicose veins are usually quite small and cause few symptoms.

## Who gets varicose veins?

A lot of studies have been done in different parts of the world, looking for possible causes of varicose veins, but the findings have varied a lot, and it is surprising how few definite answers there are.

## Sex

Among the general population in the western world, about 20 to 30 per cent (20 to 30 in 100) of women have varicose veins. Most studies have found fewer men with varicose veins (7 to 17 per cent or 7 to 17 in 100) but, in the recent Edinburgh Vein Study, 40 per cent of the men examined had varicose veins (compared with 32 per cent of the women).

## Geography and race

Studies on the incidence of varicose veins have been done in different ways, and have often concentrated on women. Nevertheless, they all seem to show that varicose veins are less common outside the countries of the western world. For example, prevalences have been found of only two per cent in rural Indian women and about five per cent for women in central and east Africa.

## Age

More people develop varicose veins as they get older – at least up to the age of about 60.

## Heredity

It is not unusual for varicose veins to 'run in the family' to some extent, but there is no well-proven genetic basis for varicose veins.

## Height and weight

Although very obese people and very tall people sometimes have particularly troublesome varicose veins, no significant correlation has ever been shown between height and varicose veins, and the evidence about obesity and varicose veins is inconsistent.

## Pregnancy

Varicose veins are more common in women who have had children, and the more pregnancies women have, the more likely they are to develop varicose veins. Varicose veins that develop in pregnancy are said to result partly from the pressure of the uterus on the veins, but the evidence for this is poor, and relaxation of the vein walls by hormones may be more important.

## Diet and bowel habit

It has been suggested that lack of fibre in the diet and sitting straining on the lavatory (rather than squatting briefly to pass a bulky stool) might predispose to varicose veins.

This idea has given rise to a lot of debate, but there is no real evidence to support it.

## Occupation and posture

A number of studies have found that varicose veins are more common in people who stand up at work – particularly those who stand still for long periods.

## Tight clothing

There has been a traditional belief that wearing tight clothes, such as corsets, might lead to varicose veins. There is some evidence that this may be true, but it is difficult to separate the wearing of corsets from the effect of increasing age.

# Why do veins become varicose?

The answer, in most cases, is that we don't really know what causes varicose veins. There are two main theories.

## 'Descending valvular incompetence'

If the valve at the top of a vein (for example, the valve at the top of the long saphenous vein in the groin)

## The changes that create varicose veins

If one valve stops working properly, this applies an abnormally high pressure on the section of vein beneath it. This pressure causes a stretching that makes the next valve down incompetent, and so on.

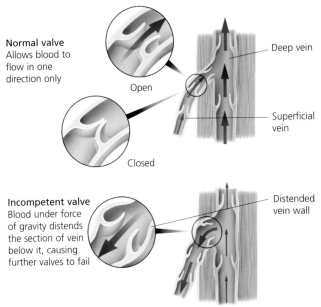

**Normal valve**
Allows blood to flow in one direction only

Open

Deep vein

Closed

Superficial vein

**Incompetent valve**
Blood under force of gravity distends the section of vein below it, causing further valves to fail

Distended vein wall

becomes 'incompetent' and stops working properly, this allows a head of pressure to distend the section of vein below it. This stretches the vein's wall, making it varicose, and this makes the next valve down incompetent, and so on down the leg.

## Weakening of the vein wall

There is some evidence that the amount of collagen (which gives strength) and the quality of the elastin (which gives elasticity) are abnormal in the leg veins of people who develop varicose veins. It is therefore possible that weakening of the vein wall is the cause of varicose veins, but not all the studies done on vein walls are in agreement about these changes.

This theory applies to 'primary varicose veins' – the usual kind that develop for no very obvious reason. A very few people get 'secondary varicose veins' as a result of deep vein thrombosis blocking the deep veins, tumours in the pelvis pressing on the leg veins or rare congenital problems (abnormal conditions present at birth) with the arteries and veins.

## What trouble do varicose veins usually cause?

Many people with varicose veins never have symptoms of any kind from them throughout their lives. When symptoms do occur, they are generally a nuisance, rather than medically serious. Only a very small proportion of people with varicose veins ever develop ulcers or other damaging problems, and there are almost always warning signs, with darkening or eczema of the skin at the ankle.

### Cosmetic embarrassment

This is by far the most common problem that varicose veins cause, and is perfectly understandable in a society that makes women want to have nice looking legs. Concern about the appearance often leads people to attribute minor symptoms in their legs to varicose veins.

### Worry about future problems

Worry about the possible dangers of having varicose veins is common, and I include it among 'symptoms' because it is often an important reason for people seeking medical advice. Doctors need to recognise and to be sensitive to these worries, which patients are often reluctant to admit.

## Aching and discomfort

Aching and heaviness of the legs are common complaints, particularly after standing up for a long time. Some people with varicose veins get itching, a feeling of heat and tenderness over their veins. All symptoms caused by varicose veins tend to be worse at the end of the day, and relieved (at least to some extent) by 'putting your feet up', although a few people find that their varicose veins are tender at night.

There are lots of reasons that people get aches and pains in their legs, apart from varicose veins. A recent large study done in Edinburgh has shown a poor association between leg symptoms and the presence of varicose veins, especially in men. Even in women, the only symptoms that correlated strongly with the presence of varicose veins were heaviness/tension, aching and itching. Restless legs, a feeling of swelling, cramps and tingling had no significant relationship with the presence of varicose veins.

This means that people with varicose veins need to realise that pains in their legs may have nothing to do with the veins, and doctors need to question patients carefully to try to work out whether their symptoms are caused by varicose veins before advising on treatment. As aching from varicose veins is usually improved by wearing good support stockings, I sometimes advise these for a trial period: this may help in deciding whether veins are the cause.

All this is made more difficult because people who hate the look of their varicose veins often blame them for any symptoms in their legs.

## Ankle swelling

Varicose veins can cause ankle swelling in a few people, as the pressure in the veins causes fluid to be squeezed out into the tissues as they stand, sit with their feet on the ground or walk about. The swelling goes away after a night in bed.

There are many other reasons for leg swelling apart from varicose veins, and even after thorough examination it is often difficult to be certain if varicose veins are the cause. It may become clear only after varicose veins have been treated by an operation, and even then the swelling can take a long time to go away.

## Varicose veins can cause more serious chronic problems

In some people abnormally high pressure in the leg veins can cause damage to the skin, and eventually lead to ulcers. This can happen as a result of varicose veins, problems in the deep veins or a combination of the two (any skin damage caused by the veins can be called venous skin problems). We do not fully understand why most people with big varicose veins never get skin trouble, whereas a few people with small varicose veins do. Venous skin damage leads to a number of different appearances.

## Venous eczema ('varicose eczema')

The first sign of trouble is often mild eczema and itchiness of the skin – usually just above the ankle. This can be just a small patch, or a larger area. It can be settled temporarily by steroid-containing creams, but in the long term they are not a safe or satisfactory treatment, because they can cause the skin to become thin and fragile. If neglected, the eczema can become very severe, with inflamed, red, scaly skin all around the lower leg.

## Skin pigmentation

This means darkening of the skin – first to a pale brown colour, and later to a dark, shiny brown appearance (see 'Lipodermatosclerosis' on page 22).

## Atrophie blanche

This French phrase is used to describe shiny white areas of skin, which are a sign of quite advanced skin damage.

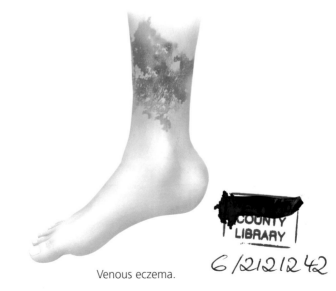

Venous eczema.

## Lipodermatosclerosis

This is the proper medical term that describes damage both to the skin ('dermato' = to do with the skin) and to the fatty layer beneath it ('lipo' = to do with fat). 'Sclerosis' means hardening and scarring. In chronic venous disease, it is not only the skin that becomes discoloured, shiny and hard; the fat beneath also becomes hard and shrinks, so that the area finishes up 'dented'.

The whole leg just above the ankle may become thinner because of hardening and shrinkage of the fatty layer. Although 'lipodermatosclerosis' is the proper medical term, I usually talk about 'skin

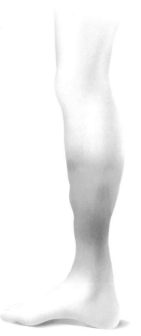

Lipodermatosclerosis.

changes', because this is rather easier to say and to understand! (See 'What is the mechanism of venous skin damage and ulceration?' on page 24).

## Ulcers (ulceration)

This means that the skin has become broken and is slow to heal. Ulcers have a raw base which may look pink and clean, or may contain yellowish 'slough'. Venous ulcers may be small or large: they may be painless or very painful, for reasons we do not understand at all.

Although there are other reasons for ulcers around the ankle, venous disease is by far the most common cause in the western world (see 'What is the mechanism of venous skin damage and ulceration?' on page 24).

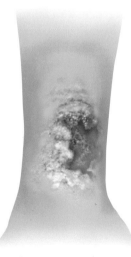

Ulceration.

## What is the mechanism of venous skin damage and ulceration?

The precise mechanism by which skin changes and ulcers develop is controversial, despite a lot of research over many years. There have been two main theories.

### The 'fibrin cuff theory'

Microscopic examination of damaged skin from the lower leg shows a 'cuff' of fibrin (one of the substances involved in blood clotting) around the capillaries. It was believed that this interfered with the passage of oxygen from the blood into the tissues. More recent research has suggested that this is unlikely to be the main cause of damage to the skin and fat.

### The 'white cell trapping' theory

White blood cells (leucocytes) contain a variety of powerful substances, which lead to inflammation, that they release when stimulated to do so. Studies on the capillaries at the ankle have shown that leucocytes become 'trapped' there when the venous pressure is high. They stick to special receptors on the capillary walls, and may then release inflammatory substances that cause tissue damage.

Over a long period this may be the cause of damage to the skin and the fatty layer beneath it.

### Putting the theories together

It may be that the fibrin cuff seen in chronically damaged skin is a long-term result of the inflammation produced by white cell trapping, rather than the cause of the trouble.

Despite considerable research, there is still a lot we do not understand about the mechanisms by which venous disease causes skin changes. Exactly why ulcers develop in the damaged area is not properly understood either, although it is clear that an injury such as knocking the leg may be the start of an ulcer.

Once the skin has become chronically damaged, it will never return to normal, and will always be prone to poor healing and the possibility of ulceration. However, treating the underlying venous problems, or using good compression stockings, will help to stop it getting worse and becoming more vulnerable (see page 39).

## KEY POINTS

- There are two systems of veins in the legs: the important deep veins and the superficial veins under the skin; it is the superficial veins that become varicose

- Normally, valves in the veins make blood flow up the leg, and the action of the muscles helps to pump it upwards

- When veins become varicose the valves often stop working properly: blood can flow the wrong way and cause a head of pressure that makes the veins bulge on standing; this head of pressure can lead to symptoms such as aching, and occasionally to skin damage

- Varicose veins are associated with increasing age, having children and western society

- We are still not sure why most varicose veins form: it may be because their valves become incompetent 'from above downwards', or because their walls become weakened

- Varicose veins can cause heaviness and aching, but there are many other causes of aches and pains in the legs; the same applies to ankle swelling

- Raised pressure in the veins as a result of incompetent valves can cause skin damage, with eczema, pigmentation (darkening) and scarring of the fat under the skin (lipodermatosclerosis); ulcers can then develop

- Despite a lot of research we cannot predict who will get skin changes and ulcers, and we are not certain how the skin damage develops

# Thrombosis, phlebitis and bleeding

## Understanding the terms

There has been a lot of confusion about the term 'thrombosis' – mostly because people have confused problems in the deep veins (deep vein thrombosis) with problems in the superficial veins (superficial thrombophlebitis). It is very important to understand the difference between these, and the different words used to describe them, which can be misleading.

## Deep vein thrombosis (DVT)

This means clotting of blood (thrombosis) in the main deep veins of the leg. The thrombosis can spread up the veins, and there is a danger that it can then detach and pass through the heart to the lungs, blocking blood vessels there (pulmonary embolism). Smaller pulmonary emboli cause chest pain and breathlessness, but big pulmonary emboli can be fatal.

DVT may cause no symptoms in the leg, or it might be painful and cause a lot of swelling. It is usually

## Deep vein thrombosis

Deep vein thrombosis (DVT) means clotting of blood in the main deep veins in the leg. The thrombosis can detach and pass to the heart and lungs where it can be fatal.

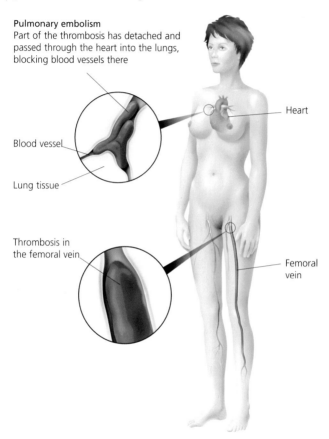

**Pulmonary embolism**
Part of the thrombosis has detached and passed through the heart into the lungs, blocking blood vessels there

Heart

Blood vessel

Lung tissue

Thrombosis in the femoral vein

Femoral vein

treated by giving anticoagulant drugs (heparin then warfarin) which prevent more blood clot forming. Natural processes in the veins then dissolve (lyse) the thrombosis, to a greater or lesser extent. The leg may return to normal, but, if veins remain blocked or if their valves are damaged by the DVT, then there can be permanent swelling of the leg, sometimes with skin changes and ulcers.

## Are varicose veins a cause of DVT?

There is no evidence that having varicose veins increases the risk of DVT in normal circumstances. The only time when varicose veins have been found to increase the chance of DVT is after major abdominal or pelvic operations.

This should not be a major worry nowadays, because surgeons take special precautions to reduce the risk of DVT at the time of major surgery.

## Venous thrombosis and air travel

People have become concerned about the risks of DVT during long air flights, following reports in the press about occasional deaths caused by fatal pulmonary embolism. For most people, the chance of DVT is minuscule and there is no good evidence that varicose veins increase this risk.

This chapter aims to reassure, to explain who may be at increased risk and to advise on possible precautions. The advice is similar for all long journeys – whether by air, coach, car or train.

### Why should long journeys cause DVT?

Sitting still allows blood to stagnate in the veins of the calf, and sitting with the legs bent (as in an economy class aircraft or coach seat) may also restrict blood flow. The longer the period of stagnation, the more likely is a thrombosis, and journeys lasting more than about five hours may pose a risk. If the blood is unusually 'thick' or 'sticky', the risk of thrombosis is greater: this can be caused by dehydration and some medical conditions.

## Who is at special risk of deep vein thrombosis?

The following increase the risk of thrombosis:

- Having had a DVT or pulmonary embolism before
- Having had a recent major operation – especially hip or knee replacement
- Severe heart disease
- Paralysis of the legs or stroke
- Malignant disease (cancer)
- Pregnancy or recent delivery of a child
- Oestrogen-containing contraceptive pills or hormone replacement therapy (HRT) – HRT is a lesser risk than the pill (progestogen-only pills should not increase the risk)
- Obesity (being overweight)
- Some blood diseases.

The risks of DVT are higher for people with more than one risk factor.

Any important increase in risk because of varicose veins is unlikely. Varicose veins have been shown to increase the risk of DVT after major abdominal operations, but not in other circumstances. People with varicose veins should not be worried about long journeys, but are well advised to consider the precautions described below.

## How large is the risk?

For people without any of the risk factors listed above the risk of DVT (even on a long-haul flight) is tiny – one in many hundreds. For people with risk factors who take no precautions against thrombosis, the risk of DVT detectable on special scans is as high as one in twenty on long-haul flights (but even then most thromboses are minor and cause no problems).

## What can be done to reduce the risk?

There is now evidence that wearing below-knee graduated compression stockings reduces the chance of DVT for people with special risk factors. As so few people without risk factors ever develop DVT or pulmonary embolism as a result of long journeys, there is no definite evidence about other measures that reduce the risk. However, based on what is well known about the causes of DVT and the successful methods of prevention used in hospital, the following are sensible precautions, particularly on long-haul flights and other journeys lasting several hours:

### Move your legs

Don't sit with your legs bent for hours on end. Stretch your legs out from time to time, and move your feet up, down and around at the ankles. Stand up to stretch the legs now and then. Stretching and moving the legs stops blood stagnating in the deep veins of the calf, and is the simplest and most effective thing you can do. Go for a walk up and down the aisle in an aeroplane; get out and walk around at rest stops during long road journeys.

### Don't get dehydrated

Drink plenty of fluid – water is ideal. Avoid excessive alcohol, which tends to cause dehydration.

### Wear compression stockings

Graduated compression stockings reduce the risk of DVT. They also help to prevent the ankle swelling which many people experience on long journeys.

- Below-knee stockings are the most comfortable kind, and seem to be just as effective as full-length stockings.

- Medical graduated compression stockings are supplied in three classes: class 1 or class 2 stockings are suitable for most people (class 3 are excessively strong for this purpose).

- Compression stockings can be prescribed by a doctor if there is a medical need. They can be bought at chemists, surgical appliance specialists, and now at some other shops, for example, in airports.

- These stockings come in a range of sizes, and your legs will need to be measured to get the right fitting.

- People who have trouble with the arteries of their legs should seek medical advice before using compression stockings.

### Deep breathing
Taking a few deep breaths from time to time may be a minor advantage in encouraging blood flow through the veins.

### Aspirin
Taking a low dose of aspirin (one standard 300 mg tablet per day) may provide a small amount of extra protection against DVT. It may be best to start taking this daily a few days before travelling.

### Anticoagulants
Special anticoagulant drugs (for example, heparin injections or warfarin by mouth) may be advisable for a few people who have medical conditions with a

particularly high risk for DVT. This kind of treatment will always be on the explicit advice of a doctor.

## Thrombophlebitis (phlebitis)

This affects the superficial veins – particularly varicose veins. The veins become inflamed, with blood clots inside them. They feel tender and hard, and the skin over them becomes inflamed. The veins and the skin may return completely to normal, but sometimes the veins remain blocked, there may be a hard area of scarring and the skin over the area may be permanently darkened.

Scanning people with phlebitis has shown that some of them develop thrombosis in the deep veins (DVT), but it is very unusual for serious DVT to develop.

### Superficial thrombophlebitis

Thrombophlebitis affects the superficial veins – particularly varicose veins.

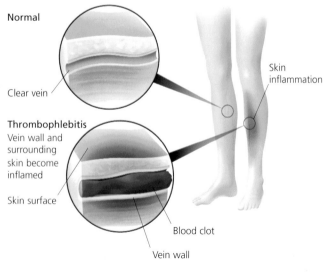

Normal

Clear vein

Skin inflammation

Thrombophlebitis
Vein wall and surrounding skin become inflamed

Skin surface

Blood clot

Vein wall

The one exception is when phlebitis spreads up the long saphenous vein (LSV) to the groin, when there is a higher risk of major DVT, and urgent treatment (tying off the LSV) may be necessary.

In most cases superficial thrombophlebitis is not serious, and simple treatment with pain-killers and surface applications (poultices or creams) helps to relieve symptoms while it settles.

Like many doctors, I prefer to use the word 'phlebitis' to avoid confusion between this condition and the more serious problem of DVT.

## Confusing other problems with phlebitis

In patients with skin changes or lipodermatosclerosis, inflammation of the skin and fat near the ankle can be mistaken for simple phlebitis. It is quite important to recognise the difference, because patients with lipodermatosclerosis need treatment to stop the problem getting worse.

## Bleeding from varicose veins

Bleeding has nothing to do with phlebitis or DVT, but this is a convenient point to mention it! Bleeding from a varicose vein is a very unusual problem, but is alarming when it happens. Bleeding generally comes from a prominent vein in the lower leg with thin damaged skin over it, and almost never from varicose veins (however large) with healthy skin over them.

The emergency treatment is to lie down, put your leg up and apply pressure to the bleeding area. If this is done then bleeding can always be controlled, because the pressure in the veins is low. If there is somebody else around to lift the leg and apply pressure, this is best. For somebody who is alone, lying on the floor, putting the leg up on a chair and leaning forward to apply pressure achieves the same effect. If restricted mobility makes this difficult, simply applying firm pressure will control the bleeding. Never use a tourniquet, which can make bleeding from veins worse.

After applying pressure for 15 minutes or so, a firm bandage should be put on, with some kind of pad over the area that has bled. Thereafter, a varicose vein operation is usually the right answer to avoid repeated bleeding.

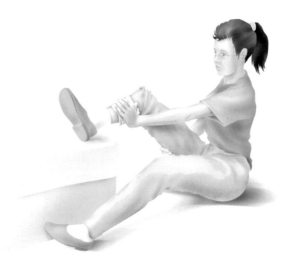

The emergency treatment for bleeding is to sit or lie down on the floor, put your leg up, for example raised on a chair, and apply pressure to the bleeding area.

## KEY POINTS

- Deep vein thrombosis (DVT) is different from phlebitis (thrombophlebitis) in varicose veins

- Having varicose veins does not seem to increase the risk of getting a DVT, except at the time of major operations

- The risk of DVT on long journeys is very small for most people, including people with varicose veins; journeys over five hours in cramped seating are those that pose a risk

- People at higher risk include those who are pregnant, obese, on the pill, or suffering from cancer, heart disease or some blood problems

- Moving the legs regularly is the most important precaution

- Other ways of reducing the small risk are to avoid dehydration, wear below-knee compression stockings and take aspirin

- Phlebitis is not normally dangerous; it seldom leads to important DVT, and does not cause blood clots to the lungs (pulmonary embolism)

- Bleeding from varicose veins is uncommon; it can always be controlled by elevation and pressure

# Simple ways of controlling symptoms

## How to control symptoms

The main methods of controlling symptoms from varicose veins are by:

- wearing compression hosiery
- avoiding prolonged standing
- elevating the legs.

Taking regular exercise and losing weight (if obese) may help. All these methods work by reducing the head of pressure in the veins of the legs.

## Elevation

This means 'putting your legs up', which removes any head of pressure from the leg veins. Ideally, the feet should be higher than the heart, but resting with the feet level with the body is perfectly adequate (for example, on a bed or couch). What is not sufficient is to put the feet on a low stool or support while sitting on a chair.

Spending long periods just sitting on a chair (with the feet on the ground) or just standing is the surest way of bringing on symptoms from varicose veins.

If you have to stand or sit for hours on end, try to get up and walk about now and then to make the calf muscle pump work. If you cannot get up, then going up and down on your toes (raising the heels) from time to time helps to pump some blood up the veins and to reduce the constant pressure on them.

## Compression

Compression of the leg can be achieved with ordinary support stockings or tights, graduated compression stockings or bandages. Compression narrows the leg veins by squeezing on them. This results in a smaller reservoir of blood in the veins, and speeds up the flow through them. It improves the efficiency of the muscle pump, and may also improve the way that fluid is filtered into the capillaries from the tissues. If swelling (oedema) is a problem, this can be reduced or prevented by good compression.

## Compression stockings
### Support stockings

Ordinary 'support stockings (or tights)' can be bought in chemists and many other shops. They give some degree of support all the way up the leg and a lot of people find that they help to reduce the discomfort caused by varicose veins.

### Graduated compression stockings

These stockings are specially made to give more compression on the lower part of the leg than higher up – the compression is 'graduated', increasing from

## How compression stockings work

Compression narrows the superficial leg veins by squeezing them. This results in a smaller volume of blood in the veins and helps the flow in the deep veins.

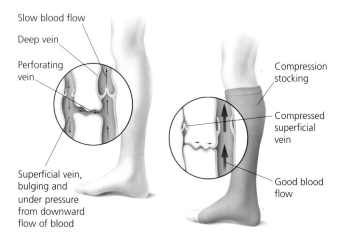

Slow blood flow

Deep vein

Perforating vein

Superficial vein, bulging and under pressure from downward flow of blood

Compression stocking

Compressed superficial vein

Good blood flow

the ankle upwards. They provide more effective compression than ordinary support stockings and tights, and are the kind that doctors prescribe (although they can be bought at chemists and surgical appliance shops).

If there are vein problems in only one leg, there is a need to wear a stocking only on that leg; there is no special need to wear a 'pair'.

Graduated compression stockings are made in different strengths and different lengths. There are three strengths of compression:

- Class 1: the least amount of compression – sufficient to relieve the symptoms of varicose veins in many people.

- Class 2: stronger. Very good support for symptoms from varicose veins, and also sufficient strength for helping to prevent progression of skin changes and recurrence of ulcers.

- Class 3: the strongest. Advised for people with skin changes, a tendency to ulcers or leg swelling that has not been adequately controlled by class 2 stockings.

The two lengths of graduated compression stockings are below-knee and above-knee stockings.

### Below-knee stockings

These are like long socks. They are usually quite sufficient for people with skin trouble, ankle swelling and symptoms below the knee only. This includes most people with varicose veins. They are generally more comfortable than above-knee stockings.

### Above-knee stockings

These need to be held up by suspenders or a special belt. They are very seldom necessary, but still often advised and prescribed by doctors. Most people find them less comfortable and less acceptable than below-knee stockings, and I only ever advise them for people who really do have symptoms above the knees.

There are a lot of different makes of graduated compression stockings, not all available on prescription. Stockings are available with open toes or closed toes (like normal socks). They are normally supplied in a brownish 'skin' colour, but some types are made in black and other colours.

These stockings come in a variety of sizes, and the circumference of the leg needs to be measured at a number of levels to select the right one. It is important

## How to put on support stockings

Support stockings are mainly intended to support the leg while up and about during the day. If you find it hard to put on a compression stocking the following advice may help.

1. Applying talc to the bare leg can make it easier to put on support stockings

2. If talc alone is not sufficient, choose an open-toed stocking and first put a plastic carrier bag over the foot

## How to put on support stockings (contd)

3. Pull the stocking on over the carrier bag. This should allow the stocking to slide over the foot more easily

4. When the stocking is on, hold it in place with one hand and remove the carrier bag through the open toe with the other hand

5. Adjust the stocking so that it is comfortable on your leg

to get stockings that are really comfortable if they are to be worn day after day. For a few people whose legs are an unusual size or shape, custom-made stockings may be necessary; these can be ordered as required.

Some people find compression stockings difficult to put on – particularly people with arthritis and restricted movement. I advise below-knee stockings with 'open toes' as the easiest; putting a plastic carrier bag over the foot, pulling the stocking on over it and then removing the bag is a good method for getting the stocking on (see pages 42–3). Some manufacturers supply 'silk stockings' to use instead of a plastic bag and it is also possible to buy other devices that help to get these tight stockings over the foot.

After several weeks of daily wear and regular washing, graduated compression stockings need to be replaced, because they lose their 'stretch', and become less effective. New stockings are usually necessary every three to four months. People who wear compression stockings each day should have two or three pairs, to allow for regular washing.

## Four-layer bandaging

Various types of compression bandage have been used in the treatment of venous problems. Over the last few years a special 'four-layer bandage' system has been convincingly shown to get most venous ulcers healed. Four-layer bandaging is done by nurses who have been specially trained – usually in clinics devoted to the treatment of venous ulcers.

It is particularly important for patients to have their leg arteries checked before putting on a four-layer bandage. If the blood flow is restricted by blocked arteries, then the pressure of a four-layer bandage can occasionally damage the skin.

## Other helpful things to do
### Exercise

Exercising the legs encourages the flow of blood up them, by the action of the muscle pump. Calf muscle exercise is particularly effective: this means any activity that moves the foot at the ankle joint. Ordinary walking exercises the calf muscles well (although spending many hours walking can make the legs feel tired and heavy). Sports, jogging and cycling are other good forms of leg exercise.

There is nothing special about 'leg exercises' done while lying down, but they are sometimes recommended for people with varicose veins, and they may suit people who find it difficult to get out and walk. Normal frequent walking is as good an exercise as any.

### Lose weight

Being overweight makes the symptoms of varicose veins worse. The box on page 46 shows approximate ideal body weight, depending on height. Getting down to an ideal body weight is likely to help with any symptoms of varicose veins.

Surgeons are particularly keen for obese patients to lose weight if they want an operation for varicose veins. Operating on obese people is rather more difficult; the risk of problems such as wound infection and deep vein thrombosis is increased, and the chance of recurrent varicose veins and further symptoms may be higher.

Having said this, surgery can usually be done relatively safely even on very obese people if there is a serious need (for example, ulcers that are failing to heal).

### Change occupation

People who work standing up all the time may find that changing to different work relieves their symptoms. Of course this may not be an easy or practical thing to do.

## What should you weigh?

- The body mass index (BMI) is a useful measure of healthy weight
- Find out your height in metres and weight in kilograms
- Calculate your BMI like this

$$BMI = \frac{\text{Your weight (kg)}}{[\text{Your height (metres)} \times \text{Your height (metres)}]}$$

$$e.g.\ 24.8 = \frac{70}{[1.68 \times 1.68]}$$

- You are recommended to try to maintain a BMI in the range 20–25
- The chart below is an easier way of estimating your BMI. Read off your height and your weight. The point where the lines cross in the chart indicates your BMI

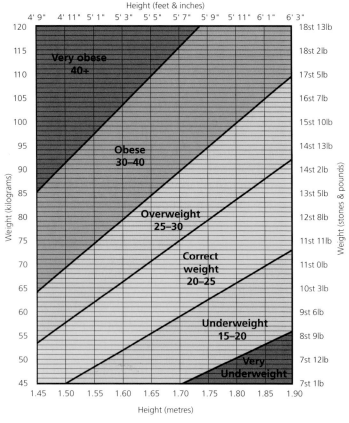

## KEY POINTS

- Compression helps symptoms and also protects the skin; ordinary support tights may be enough

- Prolonged standing or sitting with the feet down makes symptoms worse; elevating the legs usually provides some relief, but the feet must be elevated high enough

- Regular exercise helps blood flow up the leg veins; any leg muscle exercise is effective: normal frequent walking is perfectly adequate

- Losing weight is helpful for people who are overweight

# Medical assessment and investigation of varicose veins

## Seeing the doctor

Doctors the world over use the same system for working out what is wrong with patients and what it is best to do: they take a 'history', do an examination and ask for special investigations.

## Taking a history

Specialists need to ask all about the symptoms, to try to be sure which ones are likely to be caused by varicose veins.

- Exactly what symptoms is the patient getting?

- How bad are the symptoms, and are one or both legs affected? If the patient uses support stockings or tights, and they help the symptoms, this is evidence that varicose veins are likely to be the cause, and shows that the patient is sufficiently troubled to put up with the inconvenience of compression.

- Is the patient bothered a lot by the appearance of

the veins? Some people are reluctant to admit that this is a major concern, but it is important to know.

- Has the patient other worries? For example, quite a few people are concerned about what might happen to their legs in the future, particularly if older relatives have had bad trouble with varicose veins or ulcers. Reassurance may be all that is needed.

- It is helpful to know if the patient has had sclerotherapy (injection treatment) before, and absolutely vital to know if they have had an operation, because this may make further treatment rather more complex (and a duplex ultrasound scan will usually be necessary) (see page 54).

- Is there a history of deep vein thrombosis (DVT)? This is important because:
  - the deep veins may be damaged, and need to be checked before treating the varicose veins
  - there is a higher risk of DVT at the time of any operation
  - the patient may in fact only have had superficial thrombophlebitis (phlebitis) but been told that he or she had 'thrombosis'; asking 'Did you have a special X-ray or scan of the veins?' and 'Were you treated with warfarin?' may be pointers to a true DVT.

Other routine questions should include ones about general health, smoking, allergies, and regular medicines and tablets (including the contraceptive pill or hormone replacement therapy).

I always ask patients whether they have other problems with their legs (such as arthritis) and whether these limit their walking.

## Examination

Varicose veins need to be examined with the patient standing up, so that they are filled with blood. Some surgeons ask patients to stand up on a platform, so that they can examine the veins while sitting or crouching. I sit on the floor while the patient stands on the ground.

### Inspecting the legs

The surgeon looks at the leg in general (any ankle swelling or skin changes?) and then at the varicose veins, to see how many there are, how large and whereabouts they are on the limb. Varicose veins on the inner side of the thigh are almost always the result of incompetence in the long saphenous vein (LSV).

### Traditional clinical examination

Surgeons used to use no special equipment to examine varicose veins, except a tourniquet that was placed around the upper thigh with the leg elevated: the patient then stood and the tourniquet was removed while watching and feeling how the varicose veins filled with blood. This helped to show if the LSV had incompetent valves all the way up to the groin (the Trendelenburg test). Tourniquets could be placed at different levels on the legs to try to work out where incompetent valves were.

Tourniquet tests are not very accurate and are seldom used nowadays. When they are used, this is usually done with a Doppler ultrasound probe over the veins to listen to the blood flow (see below).

Another way of checking which veins with incompetent valves were putting pressure on the varicose veins lower down was by tapping on them, and feeling whether the sensation was transmitted to the fingers of the other hand, placed on varicose veins lower down. This can also be more sensitively done using Doppler ultrasound.

## Investigations
### Doppler ultrasound

This is a method that produces noises and recordings as a result of an ultrasound beam being 'shifted' in frequency by moving blood. The effect is the same as the change in sound frequency we hear standing beside a racing circuit as cars go past. As they approach, the note of the engine gets higher, and when they have gone past the note of the engine gets lower as they disappear away down the track. This change in sound frequency is called the Doppler effect (it was described by a man called Christian Doppler in the 1840s).

Doppler ultrasound can be used to produce noise from a loudspeaker as a result of blood flow: the ultrasound signal can also be shown on a screen, and recorded for sensitive analysis. A probe is placed on the skin over any artery or vein, with a small amount of special jelly on the skin surface to ensure good sound contact.

There are two crystals in the tip of the probe, one of which transmits a beam of ultrasound (at around 5–8 megahertz or MHz: 5–8 million cycles per second) into the tissues, which is reflected back to the other crystal. If everything is still in the path of the beam, then no sound is produced from the Doppler machine. However, if there is flowing blood in the path of the beam, this 'shifts' the frequency and produces a noise. The tone and character of the sound produced give information about the flow of blood.

Arteries produce a characteristic pulsatile noise, but leg veins are usually examined by squeezing the calf to produce pulses of blood flow. For example, if the Doppler probe is placed over the LSV in the thigh, and the calf is squeezed, there should be a noise as blood is pushed up the leg, but no noise when the calf is released, because the valves in the vein stop any blood flowing back down the leg. If the valves are incompetent, then blood does flow back down the vein (reflux) when the calf is released, producing a noise from the Doppler machine.

Two kinds of Doppler machine are used for varicose veins:

- hand-held Doppler
- Duplex ultrasound scanning.

## The principle of Doppler ultrasound investigation

Doppler ultrasound uses sound beams to detect moving and stationary blood. This is an important diagnostic device used to ascertain the health of veins.

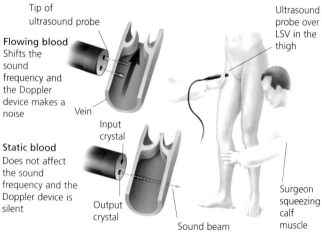

Tip of ultrasound probe

**Flowing blood** Shifts the sound frequency and the Doppler device makes a noise

Vein

Input crystal

**Static blood** Does not affect the sound frequency and the Doppler device is silent

Output crystal

Sound beam

Ultrasound probe over LSV in the thigh

Surgeon squeezing calf muscle

## Hand-held Doppler

These are small 'pocket' machines which surgeons routinely use to examine varicose veins. Hand-held Doppler examination shows:

- whether the LSV is incompetent, and at what level in the thigh

- whether there is any reflux (blood flowing back down the vein as a result of incompetent valves) behind the knee; if there is, then further investigation is needed – reflux may be in the short saphenous vein (SSV) or the deep veins

- whether there are incompetent perforating veins elsewhere in the legs

- whether the arterial supply to the leg and foot is normal.

The most important purpose of hand-held Doppler is in picking out those patients who need more detailed

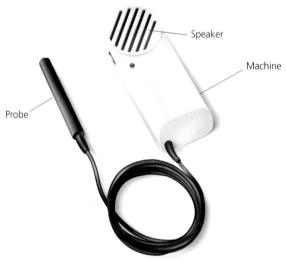

Hand-held Doppler is a small 'pocket' machine that surgeons routinely use to examine varicose veins.

examination by duplex ultrasound scanning. Hand-held Doppler examination is particularly important for the veins behind the knee, because it detects incompetent valves that would otherwise be missed.

## Duplex ultrasound scanning

Duplex means 'double' or 'two' and is the name given to larger ultrasound machines that use two kinds of ultrasound, to produce both pictures and a noise or recording. They use two kinds of ultrasound:

- The first kind produces moving pictures on a screen, as ultrasound is reflected off different tissues in the body. This is the sort of ultrasound that gives a picture of the baby inside a pregnant woman, or that is used to examine the gallbladder for gallstones.

- The second kind is Doppler ultrasound, similar to hand-held Doppler, but more sophisticated. The direction of the Doppler ultrasound beam is shown by a line on the moving picture of the tissues. In addition, a special technique is used ('pulsed' Doppler ultrasound) which allows Doppler signals to be received from any chosen depth (any point on the 'line' of the beam). By moving the direction of the beam and selecting different depths, recordings can be obtained precisely from inside any artery or vein in the ultrasound picture. This means that it is possible to show whether blood is flowing the wrong way in a superficial vein, a deep vein or both. This is not possible with hand-held Doppler.

The pictures produced by duplex ultrasound allow superficial varicose veins to be 'followed' wherever they go, to see exactly where they join the deep veins. The advanced Doppler ultrasound capabilities of duplex scanners show exactly how bad the reflux of blood through veins with incompetent valves seems to be.

Duplex ultrasound is an important modern advance in the way that we deal with varicose veins. Some surgeons have all patients with varicose veins examined by duplex ultrasound scanning. Others who are skilled in the use of hand-held Doppler use this simpler test to select those patients (less than half`) in whom extra time and expense of duplex scanning will give additional information.

There are pros and cons to each of these approaches: what matters is that all patients for whom treatment is being considered should have adequate ultrasound examination to identify clearly which veins are affected and exactly what is wrong.

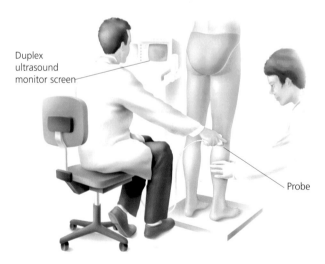

Duplex ultrasound produces pictures that allow a surgeon to follow superficial varicose veins wherever they go and accurately assess the health of the veins.

There is general agreement that duplex scanning is essential for the following:

- Any patient with reflux in the area behind the knee. This reflux may be in the SSV, the main deep (popliteal) vein or other odd veins, and only detailed pictures will provide the answer. If SSV incompetence is missed, and the patient just has LSV surgery, then varicose veins will 'come back'.

- Recurrent varicose veins after previous surgery. In particular duplex scanning shows whether there are incompetent veins in the groin that need to be dealt with at any future operation, and whether there is a length of LSV in the thigh that needs to be found and removed.

- Unusual veins, for example, varicose veins under pressure from incompetent perforating veins in various parts of the leg.

The information provided by duplex scans can be very valuable in deciding whether to operate (if all the trouble is in the deep veins, then an operation may not help) and in planning exactly which superficial veins to deal with. Duplex scans can be repeated shortly before the operation, to mark out on the skin surface exactly where difficult veins are. The accuracy of both hand-held Doppler and duplex ultrasound scanning depends on the skill of the person doing the examination.

## Other special investigations for varicose veins

### Venograms

These are X-rays that are done after injecting 'dye' (which shows up on X-ray pictures) into a vein in the foot or the groin. They can be helpful occasionally, but have largely been replaced by duplex ultrasound scanning for people with varicose veins.

### Plethysmography

This word is used for a number of different tests on the legs which help to investigate the flow of blood in the veins. They are now used only for a few uncommon problems and in research.

## KEY POINTS

- A good history of all the symptoms and details of previous treatment are essential in deciding what is best to do for varicose veins

- Examination of the leg must include some kind of Doppler ultrasound test – either hand-held Doppler by the surgeon or duplex ultrasound scanning

# When is treatment by surgery or injections necessary?

## General principles
Some kind of treatment is only strictly necessary when the skin is threatened, or when bleeding has occurred. However, other symptoms caused by varicose veins can be sufficiently troublesome for people to want treatment. This should always be a joint decision between doctor and patient.

## Cosmetic treatment
People who dislike the look of their veins may want them treated (by injections or surgery) just to get rid of them and to improve the appearance of their legs. This is quite reasonable, provided that they are clear about what treatment involves, including the risks.

Within the National Health Service, treatment of varicose veins for cosmetic reasons alone is not provided in many parts of the country.

## Aching, heaviness and itching

The decision depends on what kind of treatment would be best, and whether the patient feels that his or her symptoms are bad enough to want that treatment, with its inconvenience and risks. Surgeons need to explain to patients exactly what treatment would involve in their particular case, and whether this seems reasonable from a medical point of view.

Having been told what treatment would be possible and reasonable, it is really up to the individual patient to make up his or her mind whether the veins are troublesome enough to want them dealt with.

If people are uncertain, I suggest that they:

- take time to consider what they have been told
- read a detailed advice booklet about varicose vein surgery (or sclerotherapy)
- read a copy of the letter to their general practitioner

and then set out the pros and cons in their own case.

The decision may be particularly difficult for people with a variety of different symptoms in their legs, only some of which are definitely caused by varicose veins. It is vital that people are quite clear about the benefits that an operation is likely to offer, as well as the risks.

## Skin changes: eczema and pigmentation

Once the skin has started to become damaged some kind of treatment is advisable. For people who do not want surgery or sclerotherapy, it is quite reasonable to wear graduated compression stockings, provided that the skin problems do not worsen despite them.

Occasionally, sclerotherapy of incompetent perforating veins may be reasonable treatment. More often, surgery provides the best way of protecting the skin in the long term, if the skin changes are caused entirely by varicose veins (rather than trouble in the deep veins).

Decisions about treatment may be affected by age. For example, a young person with bad skin changes would be well advised to have an operation if this would put the veins right, whereas a very elderly person with mild skin changes is unlikely to develop ulcers and it may be reasonable to agree on no treatment at all.

If the trouble is partly in the superficial veins (which can be dealt with by an operation) and partly in the deep veins (which cannot), then the best advice may still be for an operation, followed by the regular wearing of graduated compression stockings. When there is a mixture of problems in both superficial and deep veins, decisions about surgical treatment are not straightforward.

## Ulcers

Patients with venous ulcers and varicose veins should always be considered for surgical treatment of their veins. Removal of the varicose veins may help ulcers to heal, and helps guard against further ulceration. If there are deep vein problems as well, or if an ulcer has been healed by compression in an unfit patient, then surgery may not be the best option.

## Phlebitis

What to do about treatment after an attack of phlebitis (see page 34) depends on a number of considerations:

● If the varicose veins have caused other troublesome symptoms, then the patient may want them dealt with.

- If a first attack of phlebitis was very severe, patient and surgeon may agree that an operation is best, to try to prevent another bad attack of phlebitis.

- If the affected varicose veins remain blocked off as a result of the phlebitis, then there is no need to consider removing them. They will gradually shrivel up.

- If phlebitis occurs more than once, it may be best to remove the varicose veins, to reduce the chance of further attacks.

## Bleeding

This is an alarming symptom, and can be dangerous. It is generally best to remove or inject the varicose veins, to stop it happening again. I usually remove the small area that has bled as well, so it is quite clear that the problem has really been sorted out.

## Where does the blood flow after veins have been removed?

People are often worried that, if varicose veins are removed or injected there may not be enough veins left in the leg for normal blood flow. The removal of varicose veins does not normally interfere with blood flow up the leg for two reasons:

- There are many other veins that carry the blood (particularly the deep veins).

- Blood was flowing the wrong way in the varicose veins, because their valves were not working properly.

Varicose vein operations actually improve the efficiency of the blood flow by removing damaged veins and leaving the healthy ones.

## KEY POINTS

■ For most people with varicose veins, the decision about treatment by surgery or sclerotherapy depends entirely on how troublesome the veins are

■ People with skin changes, ulcers or bleeding caused by varicose veins ought to consider some kind of treatment to reduce the chance of further trouble

■ Treatment is not essential after an attack of phlebitis, but may be best if the veins are troublesome, or if phlebitis was very bad or recurs

■ There are many veins in the legs and properly planned removal of varicose veins will leave more than enough veins for normal blood flow

# Injection treatment for varicose veins, including foam sclerotherapy

### What is injection treatment?

Injection treatment (or compression sclerotherapy) is a method of treating varicose veins by injecting a chemical substance (sclerosant) into them, which causes their walls to glue together, so that they close off and shrivel up.

The chemical substance injected into the vein works like a glue. For the glued surfaces to become firmly and permanently fixed, they must be clamped together until the glue has set: bandages or stockings are used to compress the veins and act as a 'clamp' to hold their walls together.

### 'Traditional sclerotherapy' and foam sclerotherapy

Traditional sclerotherapy uses small amounts of a sclerosant, injected into a vein in the leg with the leg elevated (to empty the veins of blood). The sclerosant enters a length of varicose vein or a cluster of veins, and seals them off. It works best for varicose veins that are not under pressure from incompetent valves higher up the leg – ideally smaller varicose veins below the knee. This 'traditional' kind of sclerotherapy has been used for years.

Foam sclerotherapy was developed in the late 1990s and has become increasingly popular. It is different from traditional sclerotherapy because the sclerosant is mixed with a small quantity of air (or other special gas) to create a foam. This foam (thousands of tiny air bubbles coated with sclerosant) spreads rapidly and widely through the veins, pushing blood out of the way and achieving better contact with the vein wall. The foam causes veins to go into spasm (shrivel up) and it is therefore more effective than ordinary sclerotherapy done without the use of foam.

## How sclerotherapy is done

Sclerotherapy is done as an outpatient (no overnight stay), either by one of the surgical team, or sometimes by another doctor or special nurse working with them who has special experience in sclerotherapy.

## Traditional sclerotherapy

For traditional sclerotherapy, the patient is often asked to stand or hang the leg over the edge of the couch to make the varicose veins easier to see. One or more fine needles, attached to small syringes of sclerosant, are introduced into the veins. The patient then lies on a couch and the leg is elevated to empty the veins before injecting sclerosant into them. Each injected area is covered with a pad, and a stocking or bandage is then applied all the way up from the foot.

## Foam sclerotherapy

For foam sclerotherapy, duplex ultrasound is normally used to identify the veins and to check that the needle or cannula is placed correctly in the chosen vein. Ultrasound is sometimes also used to follow the progress of foam through the veins, to 'milk' foam along them and to compress veins beneath the skin to reduce the passage of foam into the deeper veins.

One or more injections are given, with the leg elevated. The patient may be asked to move his or her foot up and down at the ankle after each injection, with the aim of dispersing any sclerosant that has entered the deep veins.

Compression is applied, using bandages and/or stockings, after placing pads of cottonwool, Sorbo rubber or gauze over the injected veins. These need to be left in place constantly for several days, depending on the size of the veins injected and the preference of the surgeon giving the treatment.

For larger varicose veins, compression may be advised for two to three weeks, but a week or ten days is more usual. The compression helps to ensure that the vein walls become firmly glued together so that the veins seal off well.

The exact method of doing all this varies – in particular the kinds of pads and compression that are used. Pads may be little rolls of cottonwool, gauze or Sorbo rubber. Compression may be done with a variety of bandages or with graduated compression stockings. The bandages or stockings need to be left on for two to three weeks to be sure that the vein walls have been glued together firmly.

The amount of sclerosant that can be injected at one session is limited (for example, five millilitres) so two or more sessions may be needed to get rid of all the veins. This is because larger amounts could cause side effects, through entry into the patient's general circulation.

## Traditional compression sclerotherapy

Traditional sclerotherapy involves injection of sclerosant into the target veins. This causes the walls of the veins to glue together so that they close off and shrivel up.

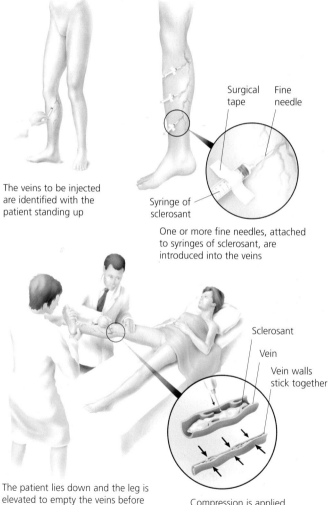

The veins to be injected are identified with the patient standing up

Surgical tape

Fine needle

Syringe of sclerosant

One or more fine needles, attached to syringes of sclerosant, are introduced into the veins

Sclerosant

Vein

Vein walls stick together

The patient lies down and the leg is elevated to empty the veins before injecting sclerosant into them

Compression is applied until the sclerosant is set

## What should you do and not do after injection treatment?
### Exercise
Much of the advice commonly given after sclerotherapy (and surgery) is not based on very good evidence, but on traditional wisdom. This applies to the usual instruction to walk briskly for at least 20 minutes after having sclerotherapy. The idea is to be sure that any sclerosant that might have got into the deep veins is pushed out of them by the action of the muscle pump.

Thereafter, regular daily activity seems sensible, avoiding standing still for long periods. If there is a need to do anything that means standing in one place for longer than about half an hour, then going for a short walk from time to time is a good idea; going up and down on the toes (raising the heels) is another way of keeping the muscle pump working when standing or sitting.

When sitting for long periods, it is probably helpful to elevate the legs, if possible. It is more important to walk about frequently than to go for a long walks, but walking long distances is also perfectly reasonable.

In general, there are no restrictions on activity and it is reasonable to pursue most sports. It is sensible to avoid very strenuous activities that cause the bandages to loosen and also contact sports that might damage the legs.

### Continuous compression
The bandages or stocking must be worn uninterruptedly, and this may mean not bathing or showering because the bandage should be kept dry. Some people get round this by showering with a large

plastic bag or bin liner over the whole leg, secured at the top with elastic or a large rubber band. Others manage a shallow bath, with the leg up on the side to keep the bandage dry. This is easier if bandages are only to knee level, and very difficult if both legs have full-length stockings or bandages. Washing between the legs on a bidet is an ideal solution.

If the bandages or stockings become loose or uncomfortable, they need to be taken off and reapplied. The sclerotherapy clinic or specialist should give you instructions about who to contact if this happens (either the clinic or a nurse working with your family doctor).

## Possible problems after sclerotherapy
### Inflammation

The sclerosant injected into the veins can cause inflammation resulting in redness and discomfort. This will settle, but if it is troublesome then it is reasonable to take pain-killers. Anti-inflammatory pain-killers such as ibuprofen may be particularly helpful, but paracetamol is often adequate. Usually any inflammation is mild and settles quite quickly. Occasionally, if it is very sore, it may be necessary for a doctor or nurse to remove the bandage or stocking and inspect the area.

### Hard, lumpy veins

If there is blood in a varicose vein when it is injected, or if blood gets into it shortly afterwards (because of inadequate compression), then the blood 'sets solid' and the vein can be felt as a hard cord, which may be tender to start with. A vein like this will usually shrivel up, but it may take a long time. This is particularly likely to happen if veins are injected behind the knee

## Foam compression sclerotherapy

Cannula

Ultrasound probe

1. The position of the vein is identified using ultrasound. The area is anaesthetised and a cannula introduced into the vein under the guidance of ultrasound

Lumen of vein

Echo from tip of needle

2. The leg is elevated to empty the vein of blood and foam is injected into the vein through the cannula

3. The location of the foam is checked using ultrasound imaging. Foam shows clearly on ultrasound

Ultrasound probe

Cannula

Ultrasound image of foam in vein

## Foam compression sclerotherapy (contd)

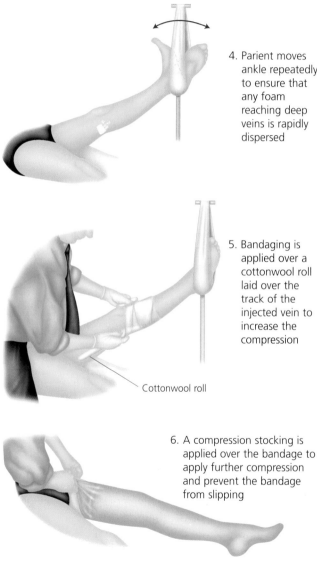

4. Parient moves ankle repeatedly to ensure that any foam reaching deep veins is rapidly dispersed

5. Bandaging is applied over a cottonwool roll laid over the track of the injected vein to increase the compression

Cottonwool roll

6. A compression stocking is applied over the bandage to apply further compression and prevent the bandage from slipping

or in the thigh, because it is quite difficult to maintain really good compression.

## Ankle swelling

A little ankle swelling may occur and is worse with prolonged standing. It will usually settle with regular walking and elevation of the leg.

## Skin damage

Rarely, sclerosant can damage the skin, even causing a small ulcer where an injection was given. If this happens the area will heal, but this may be slow and may leave a small scar.

## Brown staining

In the longer term, injections can produce brown staining of the skin in the areas where the veins were. It is unpredictable who will get brown staining and how noticeable it will be, but as many as a third of patients get some. The brown staining may fade but can be permanent.

## Thread veins

Any kind of sclerotherapy can occasionally be followed by the appearance of tiny red or blue veins in the area that was injected. This is uncommon.

## Allergic reactions

Occasionally people may be allergic to the sclerosant used to inject their veins. Any type of allergic reaction can occur – very rarely with difficulty in breathing or shock. Doctors practising sclerotherapy should always have drugs nearby to treat serious allergy.

## Deep vein thrombosis

DVT is a possible consequence of injecting varicose veins, but this is very rare. It has been a special concern during the introduction of foam sclerotherapy because small amounts of foam often enter the deep veins. However, large numbers of patients have been treated by foam sclerotherapy with only very occasional reports of DVT. Based on the information that we have, the risk of DVT is very small.

## Disturbances of vision

A few patients have had temporary disturbances of vision after foam sclerotherapy, and there has been concern that this might be a result of tiny foam bubbles entering small blood vessels in the back of the eye.

Some foam may enter the bloodstream, and it is possible that it could pass through a small 'hole in the heart' which is present in some otherwise fit people. Theoretically foam could then find its way into small arteries – for example, those in the eye or brain. The very few patients who have had visual disturbances have all rapidly recovered their full vision. The worry that air bubbles might find their way to the brain and cause a temporary or permanent stroke is a theoretical one; nevertheless it has been a matter for concern and debate – particularly as a possible side effect of treatment for a condition that is not medically serious.

## How long lasting is sclerotherapy treatment?

The result of traditional sclerotherapy may be permanent for small varicose veins, but if it is used for veins that are subject to a head of pressure from incompetent valves further up the leg, then they are more likely to come back. In the past, veins like this were often injected and came back: this is the main reason that many people regard sclerotherapy as second-rate treatment. If it is used for the right kind of varicose veins, then it can work well and give a good long-term result.

Foam sclerotherapy seems to work better than traditional sclerotherapy for larger veins and for veins that are subject to a head of pressure through incompetent valves. The results two or three years after foam sclerotherapy are similar to those of surgery, but in the longer term varicose veins may recur and require further treatment.

## What is the place of foam sclerotherapy?

At the time of writing foam sclerotherapy is finding its way into the treatment of varicose veins in the UK and surgeons are learning how best to do and use this treatment. The main skill that needs to be mastered is placing the needle or cannula in the vein using ultrasound guidance.

Around the world many surgeons have also started to use foam sclerotherapy for all kinds of varicose veins, including those that could well be treated in the long term by surgery. Foam sclerotherapy avoids an operation and a general anaesthetic, and seems to provide early results comparable to surgery. It is therefore likely to be used increasingly and it may become a common method of treatment for varicose veins.

Foam sclerotherapy seems a particularly attractive option for varicose veins that have no big connections to the deep veins of the leg, including varicose veins that have recurred after surgical treatment.

Large connections with the deep veins might be

difficult to seal off well, they might allow foam to enter the deep veins and they can be best dealt with thoroughly by surgery.

It is likely that a selective approach – offering surgery to some patients and foam sclerotherapy to others – will turn out to be best. Our knowledge of the longer-term results is not yet good enough to make definite judgements about this and more research needs to be done

Part of the reason for the rapid impact of foam sclerotherapy is that it is easy treatment to use outside hospital in private practice, so there are financial motives. As a result of this, some doctors with little previous experience of dealing with varicose veins have started to offer foam sclerotherapy: refer to 'Choosing a surgeon for your varicose veins' (page 114).

## KEY POINTS

- Traditional sclerotherapy works best for smaller varicose veins below the knee, which may be closed off permanently, but if larger veins with incompetent valves are injected they are quite likely to come back

- Foam sclerotherapy is a newer treatment that uses sclerosant mixed with air (or other gas) to form a foam of tiny bubbles, which spread widely through the varicose veins; it is normally done with the help of ultrasound scanning

- Foam sclerotherapy can successfully treat larger varicose veins, although some may recur in the longer term

- Treatment is done as an outpatient and requires compression with bandages or a stocking for two to three weeks; more than one session is often needed

- Problems after sclerotherapy are usually minor and temporary, but occasionally a little brown staining can persist

# Operations for varicose veins, including laser and radiofrequency ablation

### The objective of surgery
The aim of most operations for varicose veins is to remove the main veins with incompetent valves, which are causing a head of pressure, and then to remove all the varicose veins that can be seen. If the main superficial veins with incompetent valves are not dealt with thoroughly, then varicose veins are likely to come back.

Examination and investigation of the veins as an outpatient will have shown which main ones need to be removed. In just a few difficult cases, a further scan is needed before the operation to mark out on the skin where unusual veins need to be tied off.

### Marking the veins
Before any operation, the varicose veins all have to be marked out using an indelible felt-tip pen while the

patient is standing. This is necessary because the veins empty and can no longer be seen with a patient lying on the operating table; it also means that both surgeon and patient can be clear about all the veins that are going to be removed.

A member of the surgical team marks the veins, usually by drawing lines on each side of them (see page 81). They do this not only by looking, but also by feeling the varicose veins under the skin, trying to be sure that sections of varicose vein between the main bulges are marked: the leg finishes up looking like a 'map' before surgery.

It is important for patients to ask the surgeon about any veins that have not been marked, otherwise they will not be dealt with. I ask 'Have I marked all the veins that bother you?' to be sure. It is easy to miss occasional veins, particularly on a cold day when the patient has just arrived at hospital and has not been standing for long.

If veins cannot be dealt with at the operation (for example, thread veins) the surgeon will explain.

## Veins on the foot and around the ankle

This is a convenient point to mention varicose veins on the top of the foot and around the ankle bones, which some patients want to get rid of, but which hardly ever cause any trouble except by their appearance.

Traditionally, surgeons have been taught that treatment of these veins is both unnecessary and risky, because small nerves to the skin can be damaged (giving a numb or painful area on the foot), and there is also a tiny risk to arteries around the ankle. Some surgeons will not remove these veins, but others are prepared to do so: patients need to ask about this when treatment is first planned. I tell patients of the risk to small nerves, and leave the decision to them, removing these veins carefully if they want.

## The anaesthetic

Most varicose vein operations are done under a general anaesthetic. Epidural or spinal anaesthetics (injections in the back to make the lower half of the body numb) are possible for any operations on the legs, but most surgeons and anaesthetists favour general anaesthesia for varicose vein surgery. If just a few small veins need to be removed, then injections of local anaesthetic can be used.

Some surgeons using laser (or radiofrequency) treatment avoid general anaesthetic by injecting local anaesthetic diluted with saline around the long saphenous vein; quite large amounts of local anaesthetic may need to be injected for these operations, and some patients find this uncomfortable. The varicose veins then need to be removed by phlebectomies (see page 82) under local anaesthetic, or to be treated by foam sclerotherapy on a later occasion.

Other types of nerve block are occasionally used for varicose vein surgery, which involve injections to the main nerves passing down the legs, placing local anaesthetic around them to prevent transmission of pain messages up the nerves.

The type of anaesthetic should always be discussed with patients in the outpatient clinic when planning surgery. If a patient is worried, then it may be a help to meet the anaesthetist before the operation.

As with any operation under general anaesthetic, patients are told not to eat for about six hours beforehand, and not to drink for two or three hours, to be sure that the stomach is empty.

# How the operation is done
## Long saphenous varicose veins

The long saphenous vein (LSV) is the one that most frequently needs to be dealt with, because this is the vein that most often has incompetent valves, putting pressure on the varicose veins. The traditional and most common way of dealing with the LSV is by 'stripping' (removing it) but it is also possible to seal off the LSV using laser or radiofrequency ablation.

### Stripping the LSV

Before removing the LSV by 'stripping', it is most important that the vein be tied at the very top – where it joins the main femoral vein in the groin. An incision (two centimetres long in a very slim patient, and perhaps five centimetres long in an obese patient) is made in the skin crease of the groin, or a little above. The vein lies just to the inner side of the femoral artery (the pulse that can be felt in the groin).

The LSV is found in the fatty layer, some depth beneath the skin, and small branches joining it are all tied off and divided. The LSV is freed down to its junction with the main deep vein (the femoral vein). It is tied off next to the femoral vein (a flush 'saphenofemoral ligation') and divided, leaving a surgical clip on its lower end.

A long braided wire or fine metal rod (a 'vein stripper') is then passed down the inside of the vein to about knee level (either just below or just above the knee) and its lower end is retrieved through a small incision. It is used to remove the LSV, by tying one end of the vein to the stripper, and pulling on the other end. This used to be done by having a large 'acorn' on one end of the stripper, which was pulled down the

## Removing the long saphenous vein by 'stripping'

The long saphenous vein (LSV) is often removed because it has incompetent valves that are putting pressure on the varicose veins.

Before the operation, the varicose veins are all marked out while the patient is standing

An incision is made in the skin crease of the groin. The LSV is located and freed. A long braided wire is passed down the vein to about knee level

The wire is retrieved through a small incision at the knee. The LSV is removed by pulling the wire from one end thigh, gathering the vein against it like a concertina.

Ideally, though, the vein is 'turned inside out' (inverted) during stripping, and pulled out of one of the wounds. This is the part of the procedure that involves 'stripping' a vein – a word that is often used to describe the whole operation.

Years ago, it was normal practice to make a small incision just in front of the bone on the inside of the ankle, find the LSV there, and pass a stripper all the way up to the groin. Specialists have given this up, because it often caused damage to a nerve beside the vein (giving numbness on the inner side of the lower leg and foot) and because it was shown that the LSV was almost never varicose in the lower calf (although other veins might be).

### Laser and radiofrequency ablation of the LSV

Laser and radiofrequency are both ways of ablating (sealing off) the LSV without an incision in the groin. Under ultrasound scanning guidance a special laser fibre or a radiofrequency probe is inserted into the LSV near the knee and is advanced up to the top of the vein in the groin. Pulses of laser light or heat generated by radiofrequency are then used to seal off the vein in short lengths at a time.

### Phlebectomies (avulsions)

Having dealt with the main LSV, all the varicose veins that were marked before the operation are removed by making tiny incisions (two to three millimetres) over them, and pulling them out. This pulling out of veins is called 'phlebectomies' or 'avulsions'. Small varicose veins may cause very little bleeding when they are removed.

Huge varicose veins need some measures to stop bleeding, especially if they are in areas of lipodermatosclerosis, or if they are recurrent following previous surgery. To minimise bleeding some surgeons tie the ends of the veins as they are removed. Some apply a special tourniquet to the thigh to stop bleeding. Some simply press on the leg after removing the veins, or apply a bandage from the foot upwards to stop blood loss.

'Transilluminated powered phlebectomies' describe a technique for removing veins using a vacuum device and a powerful light. This method requires fewer (but slightly larger) incisions than standard phlebectomies. It is not widely used.

## Removing varicose veins by phlebectomy

A phlebectomy involves the removal of the varicose veins by making tiny incisions over them and pulling them out.

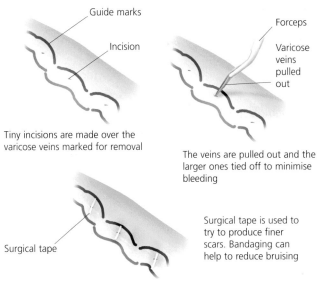

Guide marks

Incision

Tiny incisions are made over the varicose veins marked for removal

Forceps

Varicose veins pulled out

The veins are pulled out and the larger ones tied off to minimise bleeding

Surgical tape

Surgical tape is used to try to produce finer scars. Bandaging can help to reduce bruising

## Short saphenous varicose veins

If the short saphenous vein (SSV) is incompetent, it needs to be tied off just where it enters the main deep vein (the popliteal vein) a little above and behind the knee (a flush 'saphenopopliteal ligation'). The upper end of the SSV needs to be marked out on the skin by duplex scanning or by hand-held Doppler ultrasound shortly before the operation. The patient usually lies on his or her front during SSV surgery, which makes the anaesthetic just a little more complex – the patient cannot have the anaesthetic through a facemask, but requires instead some sort of special device (an endotracheal tube or laryngeal mask) to be certain that the airway is secure.

An incision (usually three to six centimetres long) is made behind the knee. The SSV is identified and dissected down to its junction with the popliteal vein, where it is tied off and divided. This is often more difficult than dealing with the LSV in the groin, because the arrangement of the veins is more variable, and there are important nerves in the area that can be damaged.

The SSV is sometimes removed by stripping (removing it) down to the ankle. It can also be dealt with by laser or radiofrequency, similar to the LSV.

## Perforator surgery

If the varicose veins are fed by perforators (veins with incompetent valves coming out through the muscles and fascia of the leg), these may need to be tied off before performing phlebectomies. This may be done through tiny phlebectomy incisions in some parts of the legs.

In the calf, the traditional operation involved tying

off incompetent perforators deep to the fascia through a long incision ('subfascial ligation of perforators' or 'Cockett's operation').

Calf perforators can also be dealt with through a telescope, passed under the fascia through small wounds: this is called SEPS ('subfascial endoscopic perforator surgery'). It is necessary only for a very small proportion of patients with leg vein problems.

## Closing the wounds

Practice varies, but most surgeons use stitches under the skin for any longer incisions (for example, in the groin and behind the knee). These stitches gradually disintegrate and do not need to be removed. The tiny phlebectomy wounds are often closed with adhesive strips, but some surgeons do not close or dress them at all because they are so small. Sometimes, fine stitches are used, which need to be removed a few days later.

It is common practice to inject long-acting local anaesthetic around wounds in the groin or behind the knee to provide pain relief in the first few hours after the operation.

## Bandages and stockings

At the end of the operation, some kind of compression is put onto the leg to reduce oozing of blood under the skin, and subsequent bruising. Crêpe or other bandages are most commonly used (sometimes with a wool layer beneath). A few surgeons put on Tubigrip or compression stockings.

## KEY POINTS

- Varicose vein operations are usually done under a general anaesthetic; a few surgeons use local anaesthetic but injections (sclerotherapy) may then be required on a later occasion

- The usual operation involves tying off the LSV in the groin, and 'stripping' it from the groin to knee level; this takes away the head of pressure on the varicose veins, and they are then removed through tiny incisions (phlebectomies)

- Laser or radiofrequency ablation of the LSV is an alternative to 'stripping' (removing) the vein, avoiding an incision in the groin; the varicose veins still need to be removed surgically through small incisions, or injected

- The wounds are often closed with stitches under the skin or adhesive strips (no stitches to be removed) and the leg is bandaged at the end of the operation

# After a varicose vein operation

## Get moving

The very first thing to realise after a varicose vein operation is that moving the legs will cause no harm. The sooner the legs get moving, the better blood flow up through the veins will be, and this helps to guard against thrombosis. It is all right to get up and walk about as soon as the immediate effects of the anaesthetic have worn off: a nurse should be sure that all is well when patients first get up.

## How much does it hurt afterwards?

People vary a lot in the amount of pain that they experience after the operation, though most experience discomfort only. As you would expect it is more uncomfortable to get up and walk after an operation on both legs than when only one leg has been dealt with. The groin wound may be uncomfortable (it is the one area of 'deep' surgery).

Laser and radiofrequency treatment avoid an incision in the groin and also avoid bruising that may occur in the thigh as a result of stripping the long saphenous vein (LSV). However, laser treatment can perforate the vein and cause bruising. For the minority of people who get problems with their groin wound or bad bruising, this can seem a significant advantage, but for most patients the overall advantage is perhaps less than many of those who promote these techniques claim.

During the first few days after the operation, 'new' aches and pains can start as bruising develops. The lower part of the inner thigh often becomes more tender, as deep bruising accumulates in the area where the LSV was stripped. The legs can become generally tender, and may be quite stiff after a lot of activity. This should not discourage people from trying to be as active as they can, but it is a good idea to take pain-killers if the legs hurt, particularly in the early days.

## Pain-killers

These will be available in hospital after the operation, and some will usually be prescribed to take home. Some people do not like the idea of taking pain-killers, but it is important to be comfortable walking about, resting and sleeping, and pain-killers are therefore a good idea during the first few days. Pain-killers that can be bought in a chemist, such as paracetamol or ibuprofen, are okay to take if the supply from the hospital runs out.

## Going home after the operation
### Day case surgery

After an operation as a day case it is usual to get up within two or three hours, and to return home after walking about a little and being checked by the hospital staff. The hospital should provide:

- written advice about the recovery and what to do in case of concern
- a note for the patient's general practitioner
- some pain-killers to take home.

If bandages need to be changed for a stocking, arrangements will be made for this.

If the operation has been done under local anaesthetic, patients may be able to get up and leave hospital very shortly afterwards.

### Inpatient surgery

Patients should get up within a few hours of the operation. People who are inpatients because they are having extensive surgery to both legs, or because they have other medical problems, may be rather slow at getting up and about to start with.

Bandages applied to the leg at the time of the operation are often changed the next day for a support stocking. Patients can go home as soon as they are sufficiently well and mobile – usually on the first day after the operation – and are given written advice and pain-killers.

## What about the wounds?

Sometimes a little blood will ooze from the wounds during the first 12 to 24 hours after the operation. The amount is usually very small and bleeding usually stops on its own.

If a wound bleeds after the patient goes home, it can almost always be stopped by pressing on the wound for ten minutes with a dressing or a pad of paper tissues. If bleeding continues after doing this twice, then it is advisable for the patient to telephone for advice or go to the hospital; this is very unusual.

The wounds may have been closed using stitches under the skin (which do not need to be removed), stitches that need to be removed or adhesive strips. The kind of stitches and dressings varies from surgeon to surgeon, and patients should always be told what to do about their wounds and when any stitches should be taken out.

Wounds in the groin can usually be washed after 48 hours, otherwise the area gets sweaty and unpleasant. The tiny phlebectomy wounds are usually closed with adhesive strips, or sometimes not dressed or closed at all because they are so small. Advice is therefore commonly given to keep them dry for 7 to 10 days.

This means not getting the legs wet in a bath or shower for that time. Some people manage to sit in a shallow bath with the operated leg up on the side (if only one leg has been dealt with). Another trick is to put one or both legs in large plastic bags with an elastic band around the top, to keep them dry in the shower! Some surgeons permit a brief shower after four or five days.

When the phlebectomy wounds are not closed, or when adhesive strips are used to close the wounds, it is often not possible to wash off all traces of antiseptic or blood from the legs at the end of the operation. All this is cleaned away during the first bath or shower at 7 to 10 days.

## Bandages and support stockings

Bandages are often changed for special support stockings the day after operation. These stockings may be worn all the time but, if they are uncomfortable at night, they can be taken off before going to bed and then put on again in the morning. They are mainly intended to support the leg while up and about during the day.

Stockings are often advised for about ten days, but there is no good evidence that they are necessary for this long. However, many people find that they make the leg more comfortable, and some people choose to wear them for longer.

## Bruising and lumpiness

Bruising and lumpiness occur because blood oozes into the spaces under the skin where the veins were removed. The larger the varicose veins, the larger the spaces that can fill with blood. Bruising is caused by blood that has 'spread out' in and around these areas, whereas lumps are formed by small collections of blood (haematoma) that clot solid and gradually harden as part of the healing process. These blood clots simply lie in the fatty layer under the skin and are not dangerous.

Surgeons try to minimise the amount of bruising and haematoma in different ways. The firm bandaging or stockings put on at the end of the operation are aimed at helping to reduce bruising. If heparin is used as a precaution against the small risk of deep vein thrombosis, then the blood clots less well and this can make bruising worse.

Bruising is common after varicose vein operations. This is sometimes quite extensive and may take a month or more to settle. It can occur particularly on the inner side of the thigh, where there may be no wounds: this is caused by old blood (haematoma) collecting in the area where the LSV was stripped. The inner part of the lower thigh may become quite tender four or five days after the operation, but it will settle.

It is common for the area under the groin wound to feel tender for a few days and thickened for a few weeks. Areas of tender lumpiness may also be felt elsewhere on the legs. This is caused by haematoma under the skin in the places where varicose veins were removed. It is not harmful and will gradually go away, but this may take several weeks.

## Walking and activity

It is important to start walking about as soon after the operation as possible. Getting up may be a little uncomfortable for the first couple of days. The whole leg may feel stiff and tender to the touch in places, but walking will cause no damage.

The aim should be to walk about every half hour or so during the day for the first week or two, and for many people this simply means getting back to their active daily routine as rapidly as possible.

The advice to 'walk three miles each day' is old-fashioned and unhelpful. Frequent walking is more important than walking a long distance, but there is nothing against going for a long walk when the legs are sufficiently comfortable.

When not walking about, it is a good idea to put the foot up – on either a couch or a bed – for the first ten days after the operation.

All the advice about frequent walking and elevation of the leg is aimed at guarding against the very small risk of thrombosis, avoiding swelling, and stopping the leg getting stiff and weak.

It is sensible to avoid violent sports while still in support stockings or bandages, and thereafter to start with some gradual training, rather than immediate competition. Swimming should be avoided until the

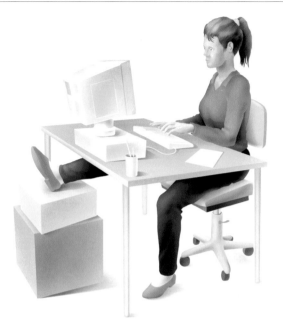

When not walking about, it is advisable to elevate the leg for the first 10 days after the operation.

support stockings or bandages have been discarded and all the wounds are dry and healed.

## Returning to work

No harm is likely to be done by people returning to work as soon as they feel able after a varicose vein operation: I have seen keen self-employed patients returning to work the next day! However, in planning likely time off, it is wise to allow two weeks for any job that involves prolonged standing or driving. It is unusual to need more than about three weeks off work after surgery to one leg, or four weeks after surgery to both legs.

## Driving a car

The most important question before driving after any operation is: 'Could you make an emergency stop without pain?' This is often about a week after surgery to one leg, or ten days after surgery to both legs. Any patient who drives an automatic car and who has had surgery to the left leg only may find that they can drive very soon afterwards! If there is any doubt or concern, then patients are best advised to check with their insurance company.

## Getting fully back to normal

The time taken to get completely back to normal varies a lot from person to person. It depends on how large and extensive the varicose veins were, and on whether the operation was on one leg or both legs. Slim people who have surgery to one leg only and who have little bruising may feel that they have recovered fully within about two or three weeks. People who are overweight, and who have had extensive bruising or surgery to both legs may take two or three months to feel that they have got over the operation completely.

Symptoms of discomfort from varicose veins tend to be noticeably better within a month or so of surgery. Swelling of the ankles may take much longer to settle. The little scars take several months to fade.

## KEY POINTS

■ It is important to get the legs moving after surgery, and to avoid prolonged standing; frequent walking is better than occasional long walks

■ There is no harm in becoming active and getting back to work quickly, but it is sensible to plan for a couple of weeks off after most varicose vein operations

■ Wearing a special stocking or bandage is usually advised for the first ten days

■ There is often a fair amount of bruising, which may take a few weeks to go away

■ There may be less discomfort after operations using laser or radiofrequency for the long saphenous vein, but varicose veins still need to be removed and this causes bruising, especially if the veins are large

# What are the risks of an operation?

**Problems and complications of varicose vein surgery**
**Discomfort**

Some pain and tenderness are normal in the first few days, but people vary a lot in how much pain they get: some have virtually no discomfort at all, while a few patients are very uncomfortable initially. Aches, twinges and areas of tenderness may all be felt in the legs for a few weeks after the operation. These will all settle down, and should not discourage people from becoming fully active as soon as they are able.

**Bruising**

Some bruising is usual and occasionally the leg becomes very bruised. This bruising may appear gradually during the first few days after the operation: it will all go away over a period of weeks. Even if the leg is 'black and blue', this should not spoil the final result of the operation. Bad bruising is more common in people whose varicose veins were large and in those who are obese.

## Lumpiness

Tender lumps under the skin are common and are caused by blood clot (haematoma) that has collected in the places where the veins were removed. Occasionally, they can be quite painful, but they are not dangerous and will gradually be absorbed by the body, disappearing over a period of several weeks.

## Infection and lymphatic problems

Infection is an occasional problem, particularly in groin wounds. It usually settles with antibiotic treatment. If the wound was closed by a stitch under the skin, this may need to be removed to allow the infection to clear up. Occasionally, an abscess may form in the groin, which needs to be opened up by an operation, and then dressed regularly until it heals.

Lymphatic vessels are tiny tubes beneath the skin that carry tissue fluid (lymph) up the lymph glands in the groin, and then on back to the bloodstream. When they are cut at an operation, they usually seal off automatically but rarely a lymphatic vessel may not seal off, producing a troublesome discharge of lymph from the groin wound, or a collection of clear lymphatic fluid which causes a lump in the groin.

Both of these usually settle down without treatment. All groin wound complications are more common in obese people and following operations that are done after previous groin surgery.

## Scarring and other blemishes

The scars are easily noticeable to start with, but will continue to fade for many months after the operation. Very occasionally, brown staining can affect the skin where the veins were removed, or areas of tiny bluish veins appear in the skin nearby, which are permanent: this is unpredictable and uncommon.

## Nerve damage

Nerves under the skin can be damaged when removing varicose veins close to them. This produces an area of numbness on the leg, which usually gets smaller over weeks or months. If varicose veins on the foot are removed, damage to small nerves is a special danger.

If a nerve lying alongside one of the main veins under the skin is damaged, then a larger area of numbness can be caused. If the nerve alongside the long saphenous vein (LSV) is damaged, numbness will result over the inner part of the lower leg and foot. If a main vein behind the knee needs to be dealt with, there is a risk to the nerve that conducts feeling from the skin on the outer part of the lower leg and foot (the sural nerve) and numbness can occur in that area. There is also a tiny danger to the main nerves that move the leg and foot when operating behind the knee.

### Will the nerve recover?

Any nerve damage recovers over a period of months if the nerve has simply been stretched or bruised, but if it has been divided then complete recovery cannot occur. Small areas of permanent numbness are quite common on the lower leg after varicose vein surgery. Radiofrequency ablation can sometimes cause areas of numbness.

If a nerve is damaged, then feelings of 'pins and needles' can occur while the nerve is recovering, and the skin in the area can also be more than usually sensitive to touch. Very occasionally, feelings like this can persist in the area of a damaged nerve, and occasional people suffer sharp shooting pains.

Persistent symptoms like these are uncommon.

Nerve damage is the most common reason that patients take legal action against surgeons after varicose vein surgery. However, damage to nerves causing numbness of the skin is a well-recognised complication of varicose vein surgery, and patients should approach the operation only if they have been given information about this risk, and have accepted the possibility of it happening.

## Deep vein thrombosis

Deep vein thrombosis (DVT) causes swelling of the leg and can result in blood clots passing to the lungs (pulmonary embolism). It is a possible complication after varicose vein surgery, but is particularly unlikely in patients who start moving their legs and walking soon after the operation. An injection of heparin may be given at the time of the operation (and sometimes afterwards) to make the blood clot less than normal. Heparin reduces the risk of DVT but may increase bruising.

The risk of thrombosis is increased in women who are taking contraceptive pills containing oestrogen, although the risk is small for operations on just one leg in women who are fit.

Surgeons will often prescribe heparin and they may discuss the pros and cons of stopping the pill for a few weeks. Getting up and about as soon as possible after the operation is particularly important for women taking the pill, and wearing antiembolism stockings also reduces the risk of DVT.

The risks are higher for operations that involve a long anaesthetic and in women who have other risk factors, such as obesity. The risk is also increased a little by taking hormone replacement therapy (HRT), but it is usual to advise patients to continue HRT while taking precautions against thrombosis.

## Leg swelling

A few people get swelling of the leg, particularly around the ankle, after varicose vein surgery. This happens particularly after operations for skin problems and for recurrent varicose veins (after a previous operation), and in people who had a tendency to leg swelling before the operation. It is caused by disturbance of the tiny lymphatic channels that drain tissue fluid from the foot and leg, and that run in the fatty layer under the skin, near the varicose veins. It may take many weeks to settle, and just occasionally people are left with some swelling in the long term.

## Damage to major arteries and deep veins

These have occurred during varicose vein surgery, but they are very rare complications, which surgeons take great pains to avoid. Surgery to repair the damage is usually done at the time of the varicose vein operation.

## Anaesthetic risks

Most varicose vein operations are performed under a general anaesthetic. General anaesthetics have some risks, which may be increased in people with chronic medical conditions, but in general they are as follows:

- Common temporary side effects (risk of 1 in 10 to 1 in 100) include bruising or pain in the area of injections, blurred vision and sickness (these can usually be treated and pass off quickly).

- Infrequent complications (risk of 1 in 100 to 1 in 10,000) include temporary breathing difficulties, muscle pains, headaches, damage to teeth, lip or tongue, sore throat and temporary difficulty speaking.

- Extremely rare and serious complications (risk of less than 1 in 10,000). These include severe allergic reactions and death, brain damage, kidney and liver failure, lung damage, permanent nerve or blood vessel damage, eye injury, and damage to the voice box or larynx. These are very rare and may depend on whether you have other serious medical conditions.

From the anaesthetic point of view varicose vein operations are generally very safe.

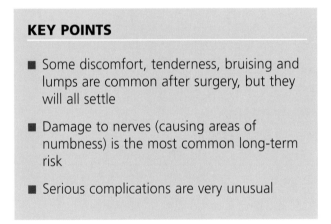

**KEY POINTS**

- Some discomfort, tenderness, bruising and lumps are common after surgery, but they will all settle

- Damage to nerves (causing areas of numbness) is the most common long-term risk

- Serious complications are very unusual

# Will the varicose veins come back?

## What is the likelihood of recurrence?

Some people develop new varicose veins during the years after a varicose vein operation, but this is less common after thorough surgery.

About one patient in five develops new varicose veins after five years and about one in four at ten years. These figures apply to people who get varicose veins again as badly as before. Larger numbers of people get just a few small varicose veins appearing as the years go by.

## Why may varicose veins recur?

There are a number of reasons for varicose veins 'coming back' after surgical treatment:

- Some veins may simply not have been removed. This is why it is important to mark the veins before surgery, and for patient and surgeon to agree exactly which veins will be removed. If there are huge numbers of veins, or if the operation is being done for skin changes or ulcers, the surgeon may explain that not all the smaller veins will be removed.

- Veins have not been tied off properly. If the long saphenous vein (LSV) or short saphenous vein (SSV) is not tied off right next to the deep veins, or if small tributaries are left untied in the groin, then these small veins can gradually enlarge and put pressure on veins lower down, leading to more varicose veins.

- The LSV has not been stripped. Surgeons have not always stripped the LSV. If it is simply tied in the groin and not stripped, the chances of further varicose veins are higher.

- New veins have grown. There is evidence that new small veins can form in the groin, even after thorough surgery. This is uncommon, but very frustrating both to surgeons and to patients when it does happen. Some surgeons have experimented with closing over where the LSV is tied off to stop this happening, but there is no proof that this is effective.

- New varicose veins form in a completely different system of veins. For example, after a good and thorough LSV operation, varicose veins can develop because either the SSV or a perforating vein has become incompetent.

- Having children, being overweight and standing continuously at work may all increase the risk of more varicose veins appearing.

The first three of these possibilities can generally be prevented by good planning and thorough surgery, but the last three cannot. Surgeons hope that with improved ultrasound methods of investigation and thorough surgery, the number of recurrent varicose veins will decrease, but there will never be a guarantee that more varicose veins will not develop.

## Recurrence after the newer treatments

We do not yet know the long-term recurrence rates after laser or radiofrequency treatment, compared with surgery. There was concern that these treatments might be followed by more frequent recurrence of varicose veins because the uppermost part of the long (or short) saphenous vein had not been dealt with so thoroughly as by surgery.

However, studies following patients for up to two or three years after treatment have not shown any important differences between these methods and surgical stripping of the LSV. There is a possibility that laser and radiofrequency might have some advantage in the long term, by avoiding growth of new veins in the groin (see above), but this has not been proved. It seems likely that the overall results will be similar, provided that each method is used in an expert way.

Foam sclerotherapy may well be followed by more frequent appearance of further varicose veins than the surgical techniques, but it can be repeated if required.

## KEY POINTS

- Many people develop just a few small varicose veins over the years after surgical treatment

- The risk of varicose veins coming back as badly as before within five years or so of surgery has been about one in five and after ten years about one in four. Modern ultrasound methods of investigating the veins before treatment may help to reduce this risk

- There are several reasons why more varicose veins can appear after an operation, but thorough surgery helps to prevent this

- Recurrence of varicose veins after laser and radiofrequency ablation is likely to be similar to stripping of the long saphenous vein over the years; more recurrences are likely after foam sclerotherapy, but this treatment can be repeated

# Thread veins and other cosmetic blemishes

## How serious are they?

A lot of people get these, and they are harmless. Most men are not bothered by them at all, but many women understandably dislike the look of them. Several different words are used to describe the different kinds of small veins:

- thread veins

- spider veins

- flares

- venous blushes (the proper medical term is 'telangiectases').

Very occasionally people get a feeling of heat or throbbing in areas of thread veins. Thread veins are also found in association with more serious problems, such as areas of skin change, but they are not the cause of such problems.

Traditionally, most doctors have said that thread veins

do not matter and cannot be treated, but increasingly clinics are being set up to deal with them. Surgeons vary greatly in their interest and expertise in treating thread veins – still only a minority have extensive experience in this area. In most places cosmetic treatment of this kind is not available on the NHS, only privately.

## What treatments are available?

The main kinds of treatment available are:

- microsclerotherapy (injections)
- laser treatment
- diathermy
- thermocoagulation.

As well as doctors, beauticians offer some of these therapies, but it is very difficult to find out about their results because they do not publish details; even among the medical profession there is remarkably little information about the detailed results of thread vein treatments.

In general, there is an impression that diathermy does not give particularly good results, but a short description is given below.

### Microsclerotherapy (microinjections)
What is it?

This treatment is similar to injection treatment for varicose veins (sclerotherapy), but the sclerosants injected into the veins are different, and the injections are done through very fine needles. By injecting one small vein, others nearby often fill up too. Doing microsclerotherapy well requires quite a lot of practice.

Doing microsclerotherapy well also requires experience. There are different types and strengths of

## Microsclerotherapy

Microsclerotherapy involves injection of sclerosant into very small veins. The vein walls stick together and the veins fade away.

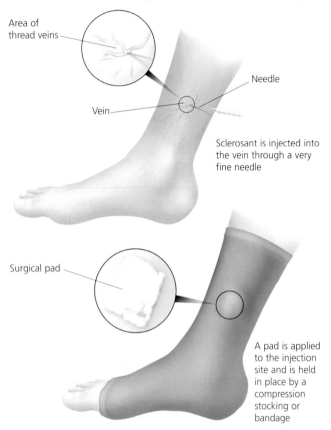

Area of thread veins

Needle

Vein

Sclerosant is injected into the vein through a very fine needle

Surgical pad

A pad is applied to the injection site and is held in place by a compression stocking or bandage

sclerosant that can be injected – some are better for larger veins and others for smaller veins.

For very tiny veins the sclerosant is injected into the vein, and the area simply pressed on for a minute or two. For larger veins, some kind of compression (with a pad, and then a stocking or bandage) is normally useful. Compression does not need to be kept on the leg for as long as after varicose vein injections, and advice varies a lot, depending on the surgeon and the size of veins – from just 24 hours to a week or more.

If there are just a few patches of thread veins, it may be possible to inject them all in a single session. If there are a lot on both legs, a number of microsclerotherapy sessions may be necessary. This is because of a need to limit the dose of sclerosant; another consideration is how much an individual can tolerate in one session.

## What happens after microsclerotherapy?

During the first couple of weeks, the injected areas can look quite inflamed and bruised, but after three or four weeks this settles, and it becomes clear how well the injections have worked. The little veins can continue to fade away for up to three months. Treatment visits are often separated by about one-month intervals.

## What are the risks?

The main risk of microsclerotherapy for thread veins is the brown staining that can follow the use of most (but not all) kinds of sclerosants. This is unpredictable and is always a small risk. Often brown staining fades over weeks or months, but in a few people it is permanent.

Occasionally, an injection can damage the skin, causing blistering or even a small ulcer, which heals leaving a scar.

## How good are the results?

The results of microsclerotherapy vary from patient to patient and are rather unpredictable. I tell anyone who is considering treatment that out of every ten people about six have a very good result and are delighted; two get fair improvement and are pleased; one has only modest improvement; and one has a poor result, possibly with some brown staining and is unhappy with the treatment.

It is very important to appreciate both this small 'failure' rate from microsclerotherapy, and also the fact that it is almost impossible to get rid of every single blemish. However, most people are pleased with the improvement in appearance that microsclerotherapy gives them.

In the months and years after a course of microsclerotherapy further thread veins may appear, which can be treated at any time.

## Laser treatment

Laser treatment is used particularly for the kind of minuscule veins that are unsuitable for sclerotherapy because they are too small to see individually and to inject. It is also used for other blemishes on the skin, such as birthmarks. Laser treatment works particularly well for tiny red thread veins on the face, but the results for veins on the legs are less predictable.

### How lasers work

A pulsed dye laser is used, which emits pulses of yellow laser light. The laser light damages the tiny blood vessels, which then gradually disappear over a few weeks. Each pulse deals with only a small area (about seven millimetres wide) at a time – it needs to be strictly targeted.

Some small areas can be treated in one session, but larger areas may require a number of visits, usually about two months apart.

### What happens during laser treatment?

Goggles need to be worn by both patient and doctor to protect the eyes against the chance of damage by the laser light. The tip of a fibreoptic laser cable is held close to the skin, and some test pulses of laser are first given to work out the best settings for the particular area of skin to be treated. The treatment is then given, and the whole session lasts about half an hour.

During laser treatment each pulse feels like the flick of a rubber band on the skin, lasting for a fraction of a second. Most patients do not find this too uncomfortable, but local anaesthetic (as a cream or an injection) can be used if necessary to make the area numb.

What happens after laser treatment: risks and results
The treated area looks bruised to start with, and it takes four to six weeks for the result of the treatment

## Laser treatment for thread veins

Laser treatment is used for the kind of minuscule veins that are too small for microsclerotherapy. The laser damages the small veins, causing them to disappear.

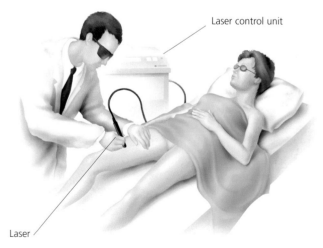

Laser control unit

Laser

to become clear. Crusting of the skin can occur after treatment, and occasionally a shallow ulcer may appear which gradually heals over.

It is important that patients should not be taking medicines that interfere with blood clotting – in particular warfarin or aspirin – just before, during or after laser treatment.

Being suntanned reduces the effectiveness of laser treatment, so it is an advantage if the area being treated is not suntanned before treatment, or for a year afterwards, because it may become permanently darker in colour (hyperpigmentation); the greatest risk of this is in the first few months. Avoiding exposure to the sun is ideal, and factor 15 or 20 sunscreen will help to protect the skin.

## Diathermy

Diathermy treatment involves passing a very low electrical current down a fine needle with its tip in a thread vein. The electricity produces heat that damages the tissue next to the needle tip, and destroys a short length of the vein. This needs to be repeated every two to three millimetres along the vein, and may cause tiny white scars in the treated area. Diathermy is generally advisable only on very small blemishes.

## Thermocoagulation

Thermocoagulation has been advertised with optimistic claims. It clearly works well for some people, but as with all thread vein treatments it is not successful for everyone. Like other methods of treating thread veins it is supported by very little good scientific information.

## KEY POINTS

■ Microsclerotherapy involves injection of thread veins through tiny needles. It will get rid of most thread veins and most people are pleased with the result, although there are a few people for whom it does not work well. Most kinds of thread veins can be dealt with by microsclerotherapy

■ Laser is best for tiny red veins that are too small to be injected; a number of sessions may be necessary over a period of several months

■ Diathermy is generally advisable only on very small blemishes

■ There is little good information about thermocoagulation

# Choosing a surgeon for your varicose veins

## How the approach to surgery has changed

In the 'old days' (before the 1990s) varicose veins were dealt with by all general surgeons, many of whom were neither particularly interested nor very expert in their treatment. Operations were often left to junior surgeons who had been trained in this 'non-specialist' approach.

To be fair, the modern methods for investigating varicose veins by ultrasound were not available, and surgeons were doing only what they had been taught. However, this old-fashioned approach often led to patients being poorly informed, having large scars and developing recurrent varicose veins, because their surgery had not been thorough.

In addition, patients had sclerotherapy when they ought to have had surgery, so their veins came back quite quickly. All this cast a shadow on the effectiveness of varicose vein treatments in many people's minds.

## Choosing a surgeon

Some general surgeons have always been enthusiastic and good at treating varicose veins. They tend to have been surgeons with a special interest in blood vessels (arteries and veins), who now form a specialist group called vascular surgeons or 'general surgeons with a vascular interest'. 'Has he or she a special interest in vascular surgery?' should be the first question to ask when choosing a surgeon to deal with varicose veins.

Even among vascular and general/vascular surgeons, there are some who are recognised as having particular interest, enthusiasm and expertise in treating varicose veins, but identifying them is more difficult. General practitioners will usually know who are the best recognised surgeons for varicose veins in your area. Ask them 'Which surgeon has a special interest in varicose veins?'.

The experience of friends who have had their varicose veins treated can be helpful in choosing a surgeon. Some pointers to a good specialist in varicose vein surgery are:

- They ask carefully about your symptoms, and how much your veins bother you.

- They use some kind of ultrasound examination.

- They ask for a duplex ultrasound scan if you have varicose veins that have come back after previous surgery.

- They explain the pros and cons of treatment.

- They either give you a choice or explain very clearly why treatment is essential (it is seldom essential except for skin changes or ulcers).

- They usually give you some written information and advice.

- Most of the scars that they make at the time of operation are very small.

If you are referred to a surgeon or surgical team who do not do most of these things, then you may want to reconsider your choice.

## New treatment or established treatment?

It is important to recognise that at the time writing (2005) varicose vein treatments are in a state of flux, with the patchy introduction of new treatments (laser, radiofrequency and foam sclerotherapy). There is no compelling evidence that one of these is 'better' than another and information about long-term results is sparse. Each has possible pros and cons, and one or other may suit particular patients.

Surgeons who claim that 'their treatment' is better than any other should be regarded with some suspicion. The place of the various treatments will become clearer with time. Few surgeons will be able to offer choice of all the possible treatments: most try to concentrate on one or two treatments that they can offer with skill and consistency.

## NHS or private care?

Treatment of varicose veins has always posed a problem for the NHS because they are just so common. Operations for them can be time-consuming (especially for recurrent varicose veins), and they are usually not a real danger to health.

For people with ulcers, skin changes, bleeding and perhaps phlebitis, the waiting time to be seen and to receive treatment should not be excessively long, because surgeons ought to give these conditions a degree of priority.

The National Institute for Health and Clinical Excellence (NICE) has produced referral guidelines for GPs about the reasons for referring people with varicose veins to hospital, and the degree of urgency with which they should be seen. However, for the great majority of people whose varicose veins are causing no physical damage, waiting times may be long. This is because the facilities (outpatient time, operating time and numbers of surgeons) are strictly limited in the NHS, and patients tend to be treated according to the medical priority of their condition.

You can ask your GP which vascular surgeon has the shortest waiting list for varicose veins: they should know because hospitals circulate this information.

If you are waiting for an outpatient treatment or for an operation and things change seriously (for example, you develop skin changes or bleeding), then your doctor should be able to arrange for you to be dealt with more quickly. If you press for earlier treatment because you do not like your veins or they are increasingly uncomfortable, the NHS is unlikely to oblige, because you would simply be 'jumping the queue' past people whose symptoms may well be as troublesome as your own.

## 'Cosmetic' varicose veins
In many parts of the country the local NHS will not fund treatment for varicose veins that are troublesome only cosmetically, and some have produced guidelines specifying other categories of varicose veins that are not eligible for treatment. This is an attempt at sensible 'rationing' of the limited NHS resources, which will always be a difficult and emotive issue.

## Cost-effectiveness of varicose vein treatments
A recent large study done in Exeter and Sheffield has shown that both surgical treatment and sclerotherapy are 'cost-effective' treatments. They improve the quality of life of people with symptoms and compare favourably with treatments used for other conditions in the NHS.

## Private treatment for varicose veins

As a result of the restrictions imposed on varicose vein treatments in the NHS in many areas, private treatment can offer considerable advantages, and may be the only way of getting your varicose veins dealt with if you have 'cosmetic' varicose veins for which your local NHS will not fund treatment. If you have private medical insurance, you are well advised to use it if you want advice or treatment for varicose veins.

The following are the main advantages of private care:

- You can see the surgeon of your choice (this might even be a surgeon who is well known for varicose veins outside your own immediate area).

- You will be dealt with personally by the consultant of your choice throughout.

- You will not have to wait long.

- You can have treatment at a time convenient to yourself.

- You can have a private room.

If you opt for private care, it is very important to be sure that you get really good specialist treatment. The 'pointers to a good specialist' shown above may be helpful; you should feel thoroughly comfortable and confident with the surgeon whom you have chosen.

## Costs of private treatment

Never feel embarrassed asking about costs. Most surgeons base their fees on the rates offered by the private medical insurance companies, so that everything should be paid for if you are fully covered by one of the leading private insurers (but note that their reimbursement levels vary a little at the present time). It is particularly important to check with your insurance company the details of your cover, especially:

- If your veins really are 'cosmetic only'. Will they pay? This applies to any varicose veins that are not causing symptoms or medical problems.

- If your veins have been operated on before. Are you fully covered?

- If you have had varicose veins for a long time, but they have only recently started to cause symptoms. From a medical point of view the problem began when the symptoms started, but occasionally insurance companies argue about this.

- If you have a policy with restrictions depending on local NHS waiting times.

Private hospitals provide 'packages' that include all costs (surgeon's fee, anaesthetist's fee and hospital charges) and your surgeon will be able to tell you about these. Remember that the consultant's fees for consultation (before and sometimes afterwards) will be additional to this.

The traditional distinction between private and NHS care may become increasingly blurred with the use of private hospitals for NHS patients under initiatives such as the 'choose and book' system.

Another recent development has been the creation of NHS 'treatment centres', which may be used for treating varicose veins. It is not yet clear how well these will work, and whether local specialists will treat patients in these centres. There is currently concern among specialists that some treatment centres may be staffed by surgeons whose training and experience is not the same as that of NHS consultants. Only time will tell.

## KEY POINTS

- Waiting times in the NHS may be long if your varicose veins are not causing real damage such as skin changes or ulcers

- NHS treatment may not be available for 'cosmetic' varicose veins

- Choose a surgeon who is a vascular specialist (preferably known for an interest in varicose veins); ask your GP and your friends; a good surgeon should inform you well, give you a choice and examine your veins by ultrasound

- Private care lets you have treatment when you want and ensures personal attention from the consultant of your choice; it means that you can get a private room, and the 'hotel' facilities of private hospitals are generally more comfortable than those of the NHS

- Always check with your medical insurance company or ask about costs of private treatment

- There may be increasing treatment of NHS patients in the private sector in the future; what NHS treatment centres will offer in the treatment of varicose veins is not yet clear

# Useful information

We have included the following organisations because, on preliminary investigation, they may be of use to the reader. However, we do not have first-hand experience of each organisation and so cannot guarantee the organisation's integrity. The reader must therefore exercise his or her own discretion and judgement when making further enquiries.

**Benefits Enquiry Line**
Freephone: 0800 882200 (8.30am–6.30pm weekdays)
Minicom: 0800 24 33 55
Website: www.dwp.gov.uk
N. Ireland: 0800 22 06 74

Government agency giving information and advice on sickness and disability benefits for people with disability and their carers.

**British Complementary Medicine Association**
PO Box 5122
Bournemouth BH8 0WG
Tel/fax: 0845 345 5977
Email: info@bcma.co.uk
Website: www.bcma.co.uk

Multi-therapy umbrella body representing organisations, clinics, colleges and independent schools, and acting as the voice of complementary medicine. Offers lists of qualified and insured practitioners of complementary medicine.

## National Institute for Health and Clinical Excellence (NICE)
MidCity Place, 71 High Holborn
London WC1V 6NA
Tel: 020 7067 5800
Fax: 020 7067 5801
Email: nice@nice.nhs.uk
Website: www.nice.org.uk

Provides national guidance on the promotion of good health and the prevention and treatment of ill-health. Patient information leaflets are available for each piece of guidance issued.

## Prodigy Website
Sowerby Centre for Health Informatics at Newcastle (SCHIN), Bede House, All Saints Business Centre
Newcastle upon Tyne NE1 2ES
Tel: 0191 243 6100
Fax: 0191 243 6101
Email: prodigy-enquiries@schin.co.uk
Website: www.prodigy.nhs.uk/PILS/indexself.asp

A website mainly for GPs giving information for patients listed by disease plus named self-help organisations.

## Vascular Surgical Society of Great Britain and Ireland

Vascular Surgical Society Office, Royal College of Surgeons of England, 35–43 Lincoln's Inn Fields
London WC2A 3PE
Tel: 020 7973 0306
Fax: 020 7430 9235
Email: office@vascularsociety.org.uk
Website: www.vascularsociety.org.uk (under construction)

Professional body representing vascular surgeons. Publishes patient information leaflets.

## Websites

### www.bbc.co.uk/conditions/varicose

Information on health matters.

### www.kingsch.nhs.uk

King's College Hospital website offering information for patients who are about to have an operation for varicose veins.

## The internet as a further source of information

After reading this book, you may feel that you would like further information on the subject. The internet is of course an excellent place to look and there are many websites with useful information about medical disorders, related charities and support groups.

For those who do not have a computer at home

some bars and cafes offer facilities for accessing the internet. These are listed in the Yellow Pages under 'Internet Bars and Cafes' and 'Internet Providers'. Your local library offers a similar facility and has staff to help you find the information that you need.

It should always be remembered, however, that the internet is unregulated and anyone is free to set up a website and add information to it. Many websites offer impartial advice and information that has been compiled and checked by qualified medical professionals. Some, on the other hand, are run by commercial organisations with the purpose of promoting their own products. Others still are run by pressure groups, some of which will provide carefully assessed and accurate information whereas others may be suggesting medications or treatments that are not supported by the medical and scientific community.

Unless you know the address of the website you want to visit – for example, www.familydoctor.co.uk – you may find the following guidelines useful when searching the internet for information.

### Search engines and other searchable sites

Google (www.google.co.uk) is the most popular search engine used in the UK, followed by Yahoo! (http://uk.yahoo.com) and MSN (www.msn.co.uk). Also popular are the search engine provided by Internet Service Providers such as Tiscali and other sites such as the BBC site (www.bbc.co.uk).

In addition to the search engines that index the whole web, there are also medical sites with search facilities, which act almost like mini-search engines, but cover only medical topics or even a particular area of medicine. Again, it is wise to look at who is responsible for compiling the information offered to ensure that it is impartial and medically accurate. The NHS Direct site (www.nhsdirect.nhs.uk) is an example of a searchable medical site.

Links to many British medical charities can be found at the Association of Medical Research Charities website (www.amrc.org.uk) and at Charity Choice (www.charitychoice.co.uk).

## Search phrases

Be specific when entering a search phrase. Searching for information on 'cancer' will return results for many different types of cancer as well as on cancer in general. You may even find sites offering astrological information. More useful results will be returned by using search phrases such as 'lung cancer' and 'treatments for lung cancer'. Both Google and Yahoo! offer an advanced search option that includes the ability to search for the exact phrase, enclosing the search phrase in quotes, that is, 'treatments for lung cancer' will have the same effect. Limiting a search to an exact phrase reduces the number of results returned but it is best to refine a search to an exact match only if you are not getting useful results with a normal search. Adding 'UK' to your search term will bring up mainly British sites, so a good phrase might be 'lung cancer' UK (don't include UK within the quotes).

Always remember the internet is international and unregulated. It holds a wealth of valuable information but individual sites may be biased, out of date or just plain wrong. Family Doctor Publications accepts no responsibility for the content of links published in this series.

# Index

# Your pages

We have included the following pages because they may help you manage your illness or condition and its treatment.

Before an appointment with a health professional, it can be useful to write down a short list of questions of things that you do not understand, so that you can make sure that you do not forget anything.

Some of the sections may not be relevant to your circumstances.

We are always pleased to receive constructive criticism or suggestions about how to improve the books. You can contact us at:

Email: familydoctor@btinternet.com
Letter: Family Doctor Publications
       PO Box 4664
       Poole
       BH15 1NN

*Thank you*

## Health-care contact details

Name:

Job title:

Place of work:


Tel:


Name:

Job title:

Place of work:


Tel:


Name:

Job title:

Place of work:


Tel:


Name:

Job title:

Place of work:


Tel:

## Significant past health events – illnesses/
## operations/investigations/treatments

| Event | Month | Year | Age (at time) |
|-------|-------|------|---------------|
|       |       |      |               |
|       |       |      |               |
|       |       |      |               |
|       |       |      |               |
|       |       |      |               |
|       |       |      |               |
|       |       |      |               |
|       |       |      |               |
|       |       |      |               |
|       |       |      |               |
|       |       |      |               |
|       |       |      |               |
|       |       |      |               |
|       |       |      |               |
|       |       |      |               |
|       |       |      |               |
|       |       |      |               |
|       |       |      |               |
|       |       |      |               |
|       |       |      |               |

## Appointments for health care

Name:

Place:

Date:

Time:

Tel:

Name:

Place:

Date:

Time:

Tel:

Name:

Place:

Date:

Time:

Tel:

Name:

Place:

Date:

Time:

Tel:

## Appointments for health care

Name:

Place:

Date:

Time:

Tel:

Name:

Place:

Date:

Time:

Tel:

Name:

Place:

Date:

Time:

Tel:

Name:

Place:

Date:

Time:

Tel:

## Current medication(s) prescribed by your doctor

Medicine name:

Purpose:

Frequency & dose:

Start date:

End date:

Medicine name:

Purpose:

Frequency & dose:

Start date:

End date:

Medicine name:

Purpose:

Frequency & dose:

Start date:

End date:

Medicine name:

Purpose:

Frequency & dose:

Start date:

End date:

## Other medicines/supplements you are taking, not prescribed by your doctor

Medicine/treatment:

Purpose:

Frequency & dose:

Start date:

End date:

Medicine/treatment:

Purpose:

Frequency & dose:

Start date:

End date:

Medicine/treatment:

Purpose:

Frequency & dose:

Start date:

End date:

Medicine/treatment:

Purpose:

Frequency & dose:

Start date:

End date:

## Questions to ask at appointments
(Note: do bear in mind that doctors work under great time
pressure, so long lists may not be helpful for either of you)

## Questions to ask at appointments
(Note: do bear in mind that doctors work under great time pressure, so long lists may not be helpful for either of you)

**Notes**

**Notes**

## Notes

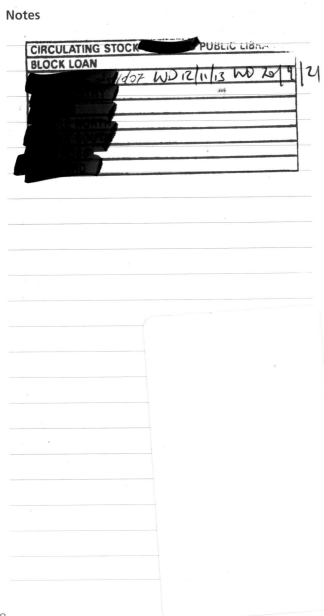